MEDICINE AND CHARITY
BEFORE THE WELFARE STATE

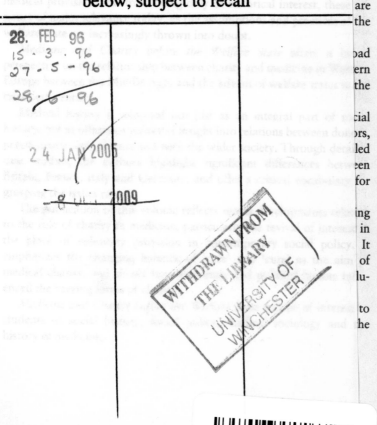

... with their overlapping roles of charities and the state in supporting medical provision ... and ... historical interest, these are ... increasingly thrown into doubt.

Medicine and Charity before the Welfare State takes a broad ... the relationship between charity and medicine in Western Europe between the sixteenth ... and the advent of welfare states in the ...

Medical history is analysed not just as an integral part of social history, but as offering an essential insight into relations between donors, philanthropists ... and ... the wider society. Through detailed case studies, the authors highlight significant differences between Britain, France, Italy, and Germany ... and ... important conclusions for comparative history.

The ... which stems reflects ... historians relating to the role of charity in medicine, particularly the revival of interest in the place of voluntary provision in the history of social policy. It emphasises the changing historiographical ... as the aim of medical charity ... in an attempt to ... medicine in its social-political ... the moving frontier of ...

Medicine and Charity explores ... will be of interest to students of social history, social policy, the ... historians and the history of medicine.

STUDIES IN THE SOCIAL HISTORY OF MEDICINE

In recent years, the social history of medicine has become recognized as a major field of historical enquiry. Aspects of health, disease, and medical care now attract the attention not only of social historians but also of researchers in a broad spectrum of historical and social science disciplines. The Society for the Social History of Medicine, founded in 1969, is an interdisciplinary body, based in Great Britain but international in membership. It exists to forward a wide-ranging view of the history of medicine, concerned equally with biological aspects of normal life, experience of and attitudes to illness, medical thought and treatment, and systems of medical care. Although frequently bearing on current issues, this interpretation of the subject makes primary reference to historical context and contemporary priorities. The intention is not to promote a sub-specialism but to conduct research according to the standards and intelligibility required of history in general. The Society publishes a journal, *Social History of Medicine*, and holds at least three conferences a year. Its series, Studies in the Social History of Medicine, does not represent publication of its proceedings, but comprises volumes on selected themes, often arising out of conferences but subsequently developed by the editors.

Jonathan Barry, Series Editor

Volumes in the series include

Life, Death, and the Elderly
Edited by Margaret Pelling and Richard M. Smith

In the Name of the Child
Edited by Roger Cooter

Reassessing Foucault
Edited by Colin Jones and Roy Porter

MEDICINE AND CHARITY BEFORE THE WELFARE STATE

Edited by
Jonathan Barry
and
Colin Jones

London and New York

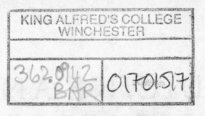
First published in 1991
by Routledge
11 New Fetter Lane, London EC4P 4EE

Simultaneously published in the USA and Canada
by Routledge
29 West 35th Street, New York, NY 10001

First published in paperback in 1994
by Routledge

Typeset by Selectmove Ltd, London
Printed and bound in Great Britain by
Mackays of Chatham PLC, Chatham, Kent

British Library Cataloguing in Publication Data
Medicine and charity before the welfare state.
1. Medicine. Sociology. History
I. Barry, Jonathan, *1956–* II. Jones, Colin, *1947–*
306. 46109

Library of Congress Cataloging in Publication Data
Medicine and charity before the welfare state / edited by Jonathan
Barry and Colin Jones.
p.   cm. — (Studies in the social history of medicine)
First published in 1991 – T.p. verso.
Includes bibliographical references and index.
1. Social medicine—Europe—History.   2. Charities, Medical—
Europe—History.   3. Europe—Social conditions.   I. Barry,
Jonathan, 1956–   .   II. Jones, Colin, 1947–   .   III. Series.
RA418.3.E85M43   1994
362.1′0425′094—dc20   93–23615
                                                                    CIP

ISBN 0–415–05741–8 (hbk)
ISBN 0–415–11136–6 (pbk)

CONTENTS

CONTENTS

CONTRIBUTORS

Donna Andrew is an Associate Professor in the Department of History, University of Guelph, Ontario, Canada. Her book *Philanthropy and Police: London Charity in the Eighteenth Century* was published in 1989. She is currently working on London debating societies 1776–1800, attacks on aristocratic vice *c.*1680–1850 and the charities of Margaret, first Countess Spencer.

Jonathan Andrews is a Research Fellow at the Wellcome Unit for the History of Medicine, University of Glasgow. He is currently engaged in a research project on Gartnavel Royal Hospital (Glasgow Royal Asylum) and psychiatry in the West of Scotland during the nineteenth century. His London University Ph.D thesis was a study of Bethlem Hospital and madness in early modern England (*Bedlam Revisited*). He has edited a short history of Gartnavel Royal (*Let There Be Light Again*) and published a number of articles on the history of psychiatry.

Jonathan Barry is a Lecturer in the Department of History and Archaeology, University of Exeter. He works on the social and cultural history of early modern England, especially provincial urban culture, and is currently revising his Ph.D thesis on Bristol for publication by Oxford University Press. He has published a number of essays, several on medical history, and edited *The Tudor and Stuart Town: A Reader* (1990) and, with Joseph Melling, *Culture in History* (1992).

David Cantor is a Wellcome Research Fellow in the Department of the History of Science, Medicine, and Technology at the Johns Hopkins University, Baltimore. He is completing a book on the relations between the State, medicine and philanthropy in twentieth-century Britain: a case study of a British medical research charity, the Arthritis and Rheumatism Council for Research.

Sandra Cavallo is a Lecturer in the Department of History and Archaeology, University of Exeter, having previously worked at the Wellcome Institute for the History of Medicine. She has published numerous articles, particularly on the history of poor relief and urban history. Her book on charity, power and gender in Turin from the sixteenth century to the end of the ancien régime is forthcoming.

Bernard Harris is Lecturer in Social Policy in the Department of Sociology and Social Policy at the University of Southampton. His main research interests lie in the social history of health and welfare in the nineteenth and twentieth centuries. He has published a number of articles on the social history of unemployment in interwar Britain and the relationship between the State and private charity in the development and implementation of social policy. He is currently preparing a book on the history of the school medical service in England and Wales between 1908 and 1974.

Colin Jones is Professor of History at Exeter University. His books include *Charity and Bienfaisance: The Treatment of the Poor in the Montpellier Region 1740–1815* (1982), *The Longman Companion to the French Revolution* (1988) and *The Charitable Imperative: Hospitals and Nursing in Ancien Régime and Revolutionary France* (1989).

Mary Lindemann is Associate Professor of History at Carnegie Mellon University and author of *Patriots and Paupers: Hamburg 1712–1830* (1990). She is currently working on a history of health and healing in northern Germany in the seventeenth and eighteenth centuries.

Hilary Marland is the author of *Medicine and Society in Wakefield and Huddersfield 1780–1870* (1987), and joint author of *'Mother and Child were Saved'. The Memoirs (1693–1740) of the Frisian Midwife Catharina Schrader* (1987). She is joint editor of *Women and Children First. International Maternal and Infant Welfare, 1870–1945* (1992) and editor of *The Art of Midwifery. Early Modern Midwives in Europe* (1993). She has also published on the history of dispensaries, the nineteenth-century medical profession, chemists and druggists, Dutch women doctors, and Dutch midwifery. Employed as Research Officer at the Institute for Medical History, Erasmus University Rotterdam, and holder of a Wellcome Research Fellowship, Dr Marland is currently working on Dutch midwives 1800–1945.

Allan Mitchell holds a Ph.D from Harvard University and is now Professor of Modern European History at the University of California,

San Diego. He is the author of five books: *Revolution in Bavaria, 1918–19* (1965); *Bismarck and the French Nation, 1848–1900* (1971); *The German Influence on France after 1870: The Formation of the French Republic* (1979); *Victors and Vanquished: The German Influence on Army and Church in France after 1870* (1984); and *The Divided Path: The German Influence on Social Reform in France after 1870* (1990).

Katharine Park is William R. Kenan, Jr Professor of History at Wellesley College, Wellesley, Massachusetts. She is the author of *Doctors and Medicine in Early Renaissance Florence* (1985) as well as a number of articles on early modern medicine and science. Her new book, on natural history and natural philosophy in the sixteenth and seventeenth centuries, will be co-authored with Lorraine J. Daston.

Miri Rubin is a Tutorial Fellow of Pembroke College, Oxford, and a University Lecturer in Medieval History at Oxford University. She is the author of *Charity and Community in Medieval Cambridge* (1987) and of *Corpus Christi: the Eucharist in Late Medieval Culture* (1991) and is currently engaged in studies of medieval society and culture and, in particular, the history of gender and the body.

Anne Summers took up her present post as Curator of Manuscripts in the British Library in 1989, after a period as Wellcome Research Fellow at the Wellcome Unit for the History of Medicine, University of Oxford. Her *Angels and Citizens: British Women as Military Nurses 1854–1914* was published by Routledge in 1988. She has been an editor of *History Workshop Journal* since 1975.

Paul Weindling is Senior Research Officer at the Wellcome Unit for the History of Medicine, University of Oxford. He has recently published *Health, Race and German Politics between National Unification and Nazism, 1870–1945* (1989). He is completing a study of European health and responses to infectious disease between the First and Second World Wars.

Stuart Woolf is Professor of History at the University of Essex. His research interests are in the social history of modern and contemporary Italy and western Europe. His publications include *A History of Italy 1700–1860* (1979), *The Poor in Western Europe in the Eighteenth and Nineteenth Centuries* (1986) and *Napoleon's Integration of Europe* (1991).

PREFACE

With one exception (Paul Weindling), the chapters are based on talks given at the annual conference of the Society for the Social History of Medicine, held at the University of Exeter, 8–10 July 1988. Both then and in their subsequent revisions, the contributors have been encouraged to develop some of the conceptual issues regarding the relationship between medicine and charity, issues which are integral to understanding the topics they are researching.

Our thanks are due to Margaret Gray and Hilary Tolley, for secretarial assistance, to Mark Davie, for assistance with Colin Jones's translation of Sandra Cavallo's chapter, to Neil Riddell, for compiling the index, and to Margaret Pelling, for her editorial help.

INTRODUCTION

Jonathan Barry and Colin Jones

The chapters in this collection offer, through a series of case studies, a critical account of the relationship between charity and medicine before the relatively recent establishment of modern welfare states. They range widely across western Europe, and cover a period from the Middle Ages to the twentieth century. They also investigate the relationship between charity and medicine from a variety of standpoints, highlighting in turn the charitable donor, the recipient, the professional physician, and the nurse. Several studies focus on hospitals, others on non-institutional forms of medical charity. Inevitably, therefore, no simple pattern is detectable. Yet despite the variety of geographical, historical and environmental settings here depicted, certain key features in the relationship between medicine and charity are strikingly persistent. This brief introduction draws out some of these regularities and recurrences, so as to suggest an agenda of issues which future historians of charity and medicine will wish to explore. Significantly too, most of these themes are of equal pertinence to continuing debates today over the place of charity in medical provision, as the assumptions and practices of the welfare state are thrown into doubt.[1]

In general terms, it might be tempting to see the role of charity since the Middle Ages declining, or at least changing fundamentally, as a consequence of the growth of the state, the economic transformations associated with industrialization, or the expanding power of medical science and the medical profession.[2] Charity, it is often assumed, will be strongest when the state is weak and voluntary provision for need is required. Charity flourishes in pre-industrial societies, characterized by the wealth of a few and poverty so extensive that it can be alleviated only by elite generosity, not remedied by public wealth. Charity follows an agenda set by the wider populace

1

rather than the medical professional, offering care rather than cure. It operates according to priorities and criteria other than those which medical knowledge might dictate. Much work on medieval and early modern Europe has suggested, for example, that spiritual concerns bulked larger in the motivations of charitable donors than material considerations.[3] Thus charity and the medical provision of the welfare state may even be viewed as polar opposites. This logical opposition is often expressed as a linear progression over time from charity to medicine, or from charity to welfare.

It is clear from this volume that the story sketched in the previous paragraph is no longer either historically accurate or conceptually satisfactory. The current rethinking of the position of modern medicine within the welfare state has confirmed the need to look afresh at the complexity of the relationships between charity and the state, charity and economic growth and charity and medical hegemony. The idea of a clear linear trend predicating the 'decline' of charity and the ascendancy of professionalized, state-backed medicine is revealed as simplistic in the extreme. As this volume demonstrates, relationships between medicine and charity have often taken a cyclical rather than a linear form, and the two have often acted as complementary rather than contradictory forces. The ideals and practices of charity have shaped much of modern medicine and have arguably played as important a part in twentieth-century medicine as before. But charity's relationship to medicine has been as problematic as it has been significant, characterized by failures, both of vision and practice, and by power struggles between groups of patrons, donors and recipients, lay and medical interests.

CHARITY AND THE STATE

The assumption that charity is an essentially private activity, to be contrasted with the public actions of government, is repeatedly thrown into question by the contributors to this volume. They show how often ostensibly private charities could be sustained by subsidies from church and state, or by exploiting the approval and patronage of the rulers to encourage other groups to donate or participate. This was as true, for example, of Renaissance Italy as of nineteenth-century France: Katharine Park shows Italian communes subsidizing hospital provision; Stuart Woolf shows Napoleon I supporting the *Société de Charité Maternelle*; Allan Mitchell shows Napoleon III offering indirect public support to mutual aid societies. The state might see many advantages in such apparently oblique methods of dealing with social problems. This approach avoided public admission that care was the *right* of the poor, rather than the gift of the rich – an important consideration for governments wedded to a liberal ideology. Such governments did not wish to see the state expand too far into individuals' affairs, lest this introduce socialist or totalitarian practices, but they were strongly influenced either by paternalistic or later by solidarist notions of the state's duties (a point seen most clearly perhaps in the French case explored by Paul Weindling and Allan Mitchell). Bernard Harris shows how the British Conservative government of 1928 followed this course, while David Cantor reconstructs the appeal of charity to cure rheumatism in the inter-war period to business people and politicians with similar attitudes. Furthermore weak or financially pressed governments might see charitable ginger-groups as excellent sources of cheap labour, willing to relieve the government of complex social problems and often possessing more detailed knowledge of local circumstances than the state could, or might want to, muster. Charities might also be able to target particular social problems which the state machinery, for administrative and political reasons, was reluctant to recognize. Often, as today, the state was prepared heavily to subsidize such bodies in return for their administrative *savoir-faire*.

Furthermore the notion of 'the state' veils the divisions that often existed within the governing elites. As Sandra Cavallo emphasizes, charity was often the arena for bitter power struggles between rival elite groups. For example, local and central government or rival political parties might support different charities or types of charity or, if one group controlled the public welfare system, another might promote 'private' charities. The story of the *policies* of charity can never be properly understood except in relation to the *politics* of public welfare.[4] Rather than supposing that the latter somehow 'replaced' the former, it seems more plausible to contend that both expanded together, with the extended patronage and power of the state being matched by the growing capabilities of charitable agencies. Weindling offers many examples of this, highlighting the growth of Church-based voluntary agencies in nineteenth-century Europe. He also reminds us that, by the nineteenth century at least, the state often extended its welfare provisions not by creating a larger bureaucracy but rather by legislating into existence welfare requirements, provision of which was left to private bodies. In these circumstances voluntary agencies, whether organized on hierarchical or mutual lines, might compete with business groups to supply public services – and often had a competitive edge in doing so. As Anne Summers demonstrates, it was religiously based organizations of nurses which established, not without painful compromises, a market position which enabled them both to satisfy and to modify the nursing needs of Victorian Britain.

CHARITY AND THE ECONOMY

This brings us to our second consideration, namely the relationship between charity and economic circumstances. It has been conventional to associate charity with the economy on two levels. In the broadest, 'macro' sense, charity has been seen as a restricted societal response to the perennial problems of poverty in pre-industrial economies which lacked the resources for – or the will to effect – a major redistribution of wealth. Although this view is not challenged directly in any of the chapters here, there is enough evidence to suggest that just as it was the richest areas and communities (notably the great cities) of pre-industrial Europe which sustained the greatest range of charities, so the growing wealth of modern Europe has expanded, rather than contracted, the aspirations of charity.

On another level, charity is usually assumed to have varied according to specific economic circumstances. As Sandra Cavallo rightly points out, however, it is not always clear whether it is boom or slump which will stimulate charity in such societies. One might hypothesize that, in the short term, slumps will activate public welfare and immediate charitable giving, while long-term institutional charity will be more likely in periods of general prosperity, in which, however, the recurrence of depressions is an ever-present threat. Mary Lindemann's analysis of Hamburg's provision for medical welfare around 1800 seems to support the latter hypothesis. As she shows, however, a slump might bring a redefinition as well as a reduction of charity. The work of Katharine Park and Miri Rubin on the effect of the Black Death in Italy and England suggests a similar conclusion: the rising wages of the poor and the financial difficulties of rentier institutions stimulated not only a diminution in charity, but also a shift of giving towards more closely defined groups.

All such generalizations, however, run the risk, identified by both

Cavallo and Rubin, of assuming too direct a relationship between demand and/or supply, created by economic conditions, and the charitable response. Instead we need, as they urge, to examine in every case how responses were mediated by the contemporary understanding of the economic situation (which might, of course, not be conceptualized in economic terms at all) and of the cultural construction of charity at that period. One of the clearest signs of this is the changing way in which 'the poor', as a category worthy of charity, were conceived. The 'language of desert' (Cavallo) is endlessly mobile, and, as Hilary Marland's work shows, often has a distinctive local edge to it.

It has become a commonplace to emphasize the dominance of moral categories such as the 'respectable poor' in the identification of groups eligible both for public relief and for charity. The innocent victims of life-cycle crises or illness, such as widows, orphans or disabled people, were often viewed as having paramount claims among this group. This was especially the case with those whose behaviour and local origins gave them an added claim to support, if only, as Cavallo suggests, as part of wider elite notions of the civic community or of family responsibilities. By contrast, adult workers, especially male heads of household, were often expected to support themselves, and if possible make provision for their illnesses, old age and dependants, through personal saving and, above all, through mutual support. Such efforts, reflecting an ideology of the independence of male heads of household shared throughout society, might be encouraged and subsidized by paternalistic elites.[5]

Many earlier examples of the realm of mutualism – 'charity between similars, not others' (Rubin) – might be given to complement Allan Mitchell's account of this phenomenon in France in the late nineteenth century. Mitchell stresses the flaws in the mutualist approach, both in its exclusion of many of the urban and rural labouring classes and in the frequent failure of mutual groups (like individual families) to provide sufficient funds to deal with economic depression, illness or other disasters. Our attention is drawn therefore to the 'potential poor' (conjunctural poor, *paupérisables*, etc.),[6] those members of the labouring classes able to live without relief or charity in good times but unable to support themselves in times of difficulty, individual or collective. The identification and classification of such people as worthy recipients of charity and the strategies adopted to keep them from falling into dependence represented a vast undertaking, and one engaged in increasingly systematically. There seems to be a close relationship between such classificatory efforts and the rise of a market economy, first in towns and then more generally, for example in sixteenth- and early seventeenth-century England, although in England it was the public poor relief system which shouldered much of the task.[7] Lindemann identifies Hamburg's decision to experiment in this direction with its growth as a port and manufacturing centre vulnerable to a world economy, within which a new 'unmoralistic' view of poverty becomes plausible. Rather than positing any necessary relationship between economic change and a particular policy, however, one should perhaps see this, as Cavallo urges, as one of a number of coexisting relief strategies, made perhaps more cogent by particular circumstances, but depending for its implementation on a range of factors affecting elite action. Certainly, as Lindemann demonstrates, the alternative model that relief should be restricted to the 'moral poor' remained powerful and staged a powerful comeback in early nineteenth-century Hamburg, just as it did in Britain at the same time.[8] Medical relief for the poor that did not entail prior descent into and acceptance of dependence, for example through the 'workhouse test', was the most notable casualty of this change.

As this suggests, medical charity was particularly sensitive to changing conceptions of the economic rationale and benefits of relief. Two crucial connections stand out in the chapters here. One of them is the notion, highlighted by Lindemann, that illness was a crucial factor in precipitating poverty among the labouring classes. The second concerns the possible contribution of medical charity to the maintenance and reproduction of the labour force. Katharine Park, for example, shows how Florentine hospitals after the Black Death were seen as helping to remedy labour shortages by returning potential labourers speedily to the work-place. David Cantor, for a much later period, brings out the way in which rheumatism was portrayed as a threat to industrial production. A linked theme, highlighted for the eighteenth and early nineteenth century by Donna Andrew and Stuart Woolf but recurring throughout this collection, is the interest in maternity, as from the eighteenth century in particular the parameters of charity have extended to embrace the child at risk.[9] Varying economic rationales opened up the potential for charitable activity and offered a long-term justification for expensive forms of intervention. Yet, as several contributors note, such medical charities were often held to represent good value for money, partly because of their long-term benefits, but partly too because they offered a very specific and closely regulated form of relief. They avoided, in particular, the charge that much charity was wasted on the deceitful. Hospital care – to take another example – could be subject to rigorous and highly public rules of admission and methods of administration so that donors could sleep peacefully abed at nights, assured that their money was being properly spent. Publicity issued by hospital boards highlighted the number of cases treated and cured, or of babies delivered safely, and thereby aimed to legitimize and sustain the charitable impulse.[10]

On the other hand, there were many points of tension between medical and socio-economic criteria for charity. For example, there was – as we shall see – a long-lasting tension over institutional versus domiciliary care. This was often associated with a debate over whether medical ends were best achieved by specifically medical means, or rather by economic and moral intervention. Should the poor be given access to medical care, whether in hospitals or at home, or were they best served by grants of money or measures to improve their conditions, or else just by sound moral and medical advice? These debates have been rendered more complex, for historians anxious to separate 'caring' from 'curing' functions, by the fact that pre-clinical medicine normally assumed that the environment, including diet and way of life, was an integral part of 'regimen'. Contemporaries were also well aware of the limited range of cases where professional medical intervention was likely to be successful. Hence the emphasis in hospitals on accidents and other conditions where surgical skills would be effective. In some cases, as Hilary Marland demonstrates for industrializing Huddersfield, these criteria might fit relatively happily, at least initially, with the economic needs of employers.

Yet a neat fit between medical and economic criteria was not always apparent. Often the medical needs either of the deserving poor or of the potential labour force stood in stark contrast with the types of medical care available. This was particularly so as regards charitable provision for so-called 'incurables'. The concern of charities for such groups has been stressed by the school of thought which maintains that charities in general, and hospitals in particular, should be seen as primarily 'caring' rather than 'curing' in function, or to put it in the harsh terms to which, since the writings of Michel Foucault, we have become accustomed, as agencies of confinement, repression and social control.[11] More generally it has been assumed that it was only in the nineteenth century that charity sought to find medical solutions, that is to cure. Several of the contributors to this collection, such as Katharine Park and Jonathan Andrews, are particularly concerned to argue that such *medical* charity was indeed available long before the so-called 'medicalization' of hospitals in the late eighteenth or nineteenth century.[12] The studies of Park and Andrews indicate that curing was an important priority for many charities long before the alleged 'birth of the clinic' and that donors, medical practitioners and, as far as can be judged, patients, often shared beliefs and hopes of cure. Criteria for admission often excluded the incurable or those unlikely to be relieved, while a record of success was an important part of the propaganda of charity. Indeed Marland suggests that a desire to avoid the high mortality rate associated with accident cases led to a gradual shift in Huddersfield's infirmary policy. The debate between hospital and domiciliary care, for example in infant care, centred on accusations about medical standards and mortality levels.

Late medieval and Renaissance Italy had clearly already moved beyond a stage in which hospitals were limited to caring for incurable cases, and other countries developed during the early modern period a range of infirmaries with a curative function. Yet, as today, medical relief often found itself concerned with the mass of chronic illness, infirmity and incurable mental and physical illnesses which contributed so much to poverty. A great deal of charitable effort, supplementing public relief, was devoted to meeting these needs. Here we need to be sensitive, as Rubin and others indicate, to the changing functions of institutions over time, as they adjusted their objects of charity. We also need to be aware of the creeping effects on charities of chronic cases, which could easily come to monopolize beds or eat up funds intended for a succession of rapidly cured cases. Of course, we should also not accept too easily those definitions of medical charity which deny the title 'medical' to care of such patients, a tendency often associated with the downgrading of the nursing aspect of charitable care. In line with the best recent work on the history of medical practice, it will surely be more productive to widen as far as possible our conception of 'medical relief' or therapy, rather than Whiggishly projecting back narrow definitions based either on our own standards of what constitutes medicine or restricting the term to medical care provided by a tightly defined medical profession.[13]

CHARITY AND THE MEDICAL PROFESSION

Although the question of the relationship between charity and medical practitioners should properly be asked concerning all the occupations providing medical care to charities – and as Summers reminds us, there is a whole gender issue here waiting to be fully explored[14] – it is generally asked chiefly about qualified medical men. What part did their changing ideas about the potential of medicine, their professional interests and their political and social ideals play in the development of charity? Was charity a sphere in which the laity controlled medicine, or was the exploitation the other way round? As might be expected, the chapters here suggest a complex, often paradoxical answer to these questions.

Charities could offer important opportunities to the medical profession, both to establish new types of medical care and to forge individual and collective reputations. Marland outlines the advantages to medical practitioners of a voluntary hospital position and shows how the changing medical interests of the profession might lead to a gradual shift in the types of care offered. Her work echoes findings both here and elsewhere which suggest that, whatever the situation when an institution or charity was established, over time the medical profession might come to exercise a dominant role. Medical practitioners were also interested in establishing new charities to support medical work outside the existing patterns both of charity and of medical prestige.[15] Weindling and Cantor both emphasize the role of charity in modern medical research. In many ways the Florentine hospitals described by Park form an earlier analogue, while Andrews reminds us of the pioneering, if to us misconceived, work on the treatment of the insane tried out by various Bethlem doctors. Charity cases (at least those in the English voluntary hospitals) were perhaps the first to be treated as patients in the modern sense, since in treating them doctors were freed from the social and economic restraints which made their relations with the rest of laity relatively reciprocal.[16] Furthermore, as Weindling notes, it suited the self-image of the medical profession, first as a body of gentlemen and then as a liberal profession, to support medical charities which reinforced this image of their role and which protected them from having to act as the paid agents of the state. Finally, as Marland indicates, many of these medical men came from the same social background and shared the political attitudes of the laity running the charities in which they practised.

On the other hand, working in charities dependent on lay support and run by lay administrators posed a number of problems for medical practitioners. As we have seen, there could be tensions between different views of whom the charity should serve and how. Medical staff might resent lay rules and oversight, while in cases where they were paid, such as by Mitchell's mutual societies, they might clash on the level of remuneration. Medical men, like the nurses Summers discusses, might also wish to provide more expensive care than the laity were prepared to accept, or than the funds of charities (often highly precarious) would allow. On the other hand, medical men had a vested interest in ensuring that charitable medical provision did not become too easy or attractive an alternative to paying for their services in the open market. Hence they, too, would wish to operate strict admission policies keeping out those, such as the labouring poor, who might form part of their clientele in normal years. Alternatively they might support schemes for mutual help, medical insurance or even state collective action which would offer medical practitioners a broader and less precarious basis on which to offer their services to the mass of the population. In practice, these alternatives would probably, at any one time, each have their appeal to particular groups of medical practitioners, depending in part on their career position or medical specialty, and in part on their broader socio-political outlook.

The same tensions marked the debate between institutional and domiciliary provision of medical charity. Both lay and medical groups could identify advantages in removing the poor from their homes into hospitals, subject to stricter controls, and also in leaving them in their homes. Debates raged over which was cheaper and more efficacious. Most historical attention has focused on the hospitals, but this collection should serve to remind us of the potential strengths of the domiciliary model. As Summers stresses, both lay donors and providers of care saw visiting the sick at home as the most direct way of affecting the life-styles of the poor, whether medically or morally, and here medical charity (such as district nursing) borrowed many of its assumptions and techniques from religious practices, often across the confessional divide. Even if current historiography is dubious of the characterization of hospitals as 'gateways of death' or 'total institutions',[17] they stood outside the normal experience of pre-nineteenth-century society, being associated with the loss of a household position, and increasingly with workhouses. Their depressing psychological impact should not be underestimated.

A final point arises from this: the need to study medical charity, not only in the context of other forms of medical relief and other types of charity, but also in its broader social context. For example, the origins of modern nursing lie in Victorian Christianity, Summers suggests, more than in medical technology and hospital organization. Cavallo may be correct to suggest that religious factors have been given due weight in medieval and early modern studies, but their modern impact deserves further research. More generally, the studies collected here throw a great deal of light on urban conditions at various times, but leave the nature of rural experience, still the commonplace until recently, largely unexplored. It may indeed be that new forms of charity have generally been forged in the urban setting, but one conclusion from this collection is surely the need to examine the changing practices and meaning of charity as it adapts to new contexts. So both the urban origins and the later rural appropriation of charities need examination. In addition, much more might be said about the role of the family and household formation in shaping the context and assumptions of charity. This consideration takes on particular force if we take the step, largely neglected here, of shifting our attention from the providers of charity to its recipients, and examine how and why the poor wanted and used charity.[18] Mounting evidence suggests that this owed most to the shifting household circumstances of the poor, and that they often used charity in ways not intended by the charitable.[19] For the recipient, as for the donors, charity had its benefits and disadvantages, measured not solely in economic terms but also in broader social and cultural terms. We should also not forget that, in certain circumstances, the recipients of charity might themselves be potential donors. Hence the importance of including mutualism as a category of charity, since it appealed to many of the same notions about the worth of giving as other more hierarchical forms of charity. More broadly, the state itself, as the beneficiary of public funds, can be seen as an important agent of the charitable feelings of the nation, pursued collectively. If the essays collected here undermine any simple distinction between voluntary and state provision for medical welfare, they leave open the historical perspective which sees the welfare state not as a recent aberration but a recurring and compelling option.[20]

NOTES

1 Some markers on contemporary debates appear in R. Haveman, B. Wolfe and V. Halberstadt, 'The European welfare state in transition', in J. L. Parker (ed.) *Perspectives on the Reagan Years*, Washington, DC, 1986; and J. Krieger, 'Social policy in the age of Reagan and Thatcher', *Socialist Register 1987*, London, 1987. Two collections of essays in comparative history are: P. Flora and A. J. Heidenheimer (eds) *The Development of Welfare States in Western Europe*, New Brunswick, NJ, and London, 1981; W. J. Mommsen and W. Mock (eds) *The Emergence of the Welfare State in Britain and Germany 1850–1950*, London, 1981.

2 In his thoughtful and incisive study, *In Care of the State: Health Care, Education and Welfare in Europe and the USA in the Modern Era*, Oxford, 1988, A. de Swaan, for example, posits a long-term shift 'from charity to social consciousness' (p. 252). Similar views are detectable too in C. Lis and H. Soly, *Poverty and Capitalism in Pre-Industrial Europe*, London, 1982. A long-term case study sensitive to all these issues is provided by J. V. Pickstone, *Medicine and Industrial Society: A History of Hospital Development in Manchester and its Region, 1752–1946*, Manchester, 1985.

3 B. Tierney, *Medieval Poor Law: A Sketch of Canonical Theory and its Application in England*, Berkeley, Calif., 1959; C. Jones, *The Charitable Imperative: Hospitals and Nursing in Ancien Régime and Revolutionary France*, London, 1989; W. J. Sheils (ed.) *The Church and Healing*, Studies in Church History, vol. 19, 1982.

4 A theme further explored in L. Granshaw and R. Porter (eds) *The Hospital in History*, London, 1989.

5 This is an important theme developed in S.J. Woolf, *The Poor in Western Europe in the Eighteenth and Nineteenth Centuries*, London and New York, 1986.

6 For these ideas, see esp. J. P. Gutton, *La Société et les pauvres: l'exemple de la généralité de Lyon (1534–1789)*, Paris, 1971; and Gutton, *La Société et les pauvres en Europe (XVIe.–XVIIIe. siècles)*, Paris, 1974.

7 P. Slack, *Poverty and Policy in Tudor and Stuart England*, London, 1988; M. Pelling, 'Healing the sick poor: social policy and disability in Norwich 1550–1640', *Medical History*, 1985, vol. 29.

8 G. Himmelfarb, *The Idea of Poverty*, London, 1984; M. W. Flinn, 'Medical services under the new Poor Law', in D. Fraser (ed.) *The New Poor Law in the Nineteenth Century*, London, 1984; I. Loudon, *Medical Care and the General Practitioner*, Oxford, 1986, pp. 228–48.

9 E. Seidler, 'An historical survey of children's hospitals', in Granshaw and Porter, op. cit. For earlier interest see M. Pelling, 'Child health as a social value in early modern England', *Social History of Medicine*, 1988, vol. 1; M. Laget, *Naissance: L'accouchement avant l'âge de la clinique*, Paris, 1982.

10 R. Porter, 'The gift relation: philanthropy and provincial hospitals in eighteenth-century England', in Granshaw and Porter, op. cit., pp. 156–7.

11 See esp. M. Foucault *et al.*, *Les Machines à guérir: aux origines de l'hôpital moderne*, Paris, 1979; M. Foucault, *The Birth of the Clinic: An Archaeology of Medical Perception*, London, 1974; G. B. Risse, *Hospital Life in Enlightenment Scotland: Care and Teaching at the Royal Infirmary of Edinburgh*, Cambridge, 1986.

12 The influence, alternately stimulating and baneful, has been very notable in this area. Besides Foucault's works cited in note 11, see esp. his *Folie et déraison: histoire de la folie à l'âge classique*, Paris, 1961 (abridged as *Madness and Civilisation*, New York, 1965), and *Discipline and Punish: The Birth of the Prison*, London, 1979.

13 P. Corsi and P. Weindling (eds) *Information Sources in the History of Science and Medicine*, London, 1983; M. Pelling, 'Medical practice in early modern England: trade or profession?', in W. Prest (ed.) *The Professions in Early Modern England*, London, 1987; M. Ramsey, *Professional and Popular Medicine in France 1770–1830*, Cambridge, 1988.

14 See for example for France: J. Leonard, 'Women, religion and medicine', in R. Forster and O. Ranum (eds) *Medicine and Society in France: Selections from the Annales*, Baltimore, Md and London, 1980; J. Gélis, *La Sage-femme ou le médecin: une nouvelle conception de la vie*, Paris, 1988; C. Jones, 'Sisters of Charity and the ailing poor', *Social History of Medicine*, 1989, vol. 2.

15 M. Fissell, 'The physic of charity: health and welfare in the West Country, 1690–1834', Ph.D thesis, University of Pennsylvania, 1988; L. Granshaw, '"Fame and fortune by means of bricks and mortar": the medical profession and specialist hospitals in Britain, 1800–1948', in Granshaw and Porter, op. cit.

16 Fissell, op. cit.; G. Risse, 'Hospital history: new sources and methods', in R. Porter and A. Wear (eds) *Problems and Methods in the History of Medicine*, London, 1987. In France, the same role was played by the sick soldier: see Jones, *Charitable Imperative*, pp. 18–19, 209 ff.

17 The 'gateway to death' literature is surveyed, particularly for France, in Jones, *Charitable Imperative*, pp. 48–55. See too J. Woodward, *To Do the Sick No Harm: A Study of the British Voluntary Hospital System to 1875*, London, 1974; and for Italy, see K. Park, Chapter 2 in this volume. An excellent critique of the 'total institution' view of hospitals is offered by O. Faure, *Genèse de l'hôpital moderne: Les hospices civils de Lyon de 1802 à 1845*, Lyon, 1982.

18 For the inclusion in medical history of the patient's view see R. Porter (ed.) *Patients and Practitioners: Lay Perceptions of Medicine in Pre-Industrial Societies*, Cambridge, 1985.

19 See esp. Woolf, op. cit.; M. Fissell, 'The "sick and drooping poor" in eighteenth-century Bristol and its region', *Social History of Medicine*, 1989, vol. 2; J. Henderson (ed.) 'Charity and the poor in medieval and Renaissance Europe', *Continuity and Change*, 1988, vol. 3.

20 De Swaan, op. cit.

1

IMAGINING MEDIEVAL HOSPITALS

Considerations on the cultural meaning of institutional change

Miri Rubin

Some of us, social historians interested in poverty and its relief in the medieval world, have been attracted in recent years to the study of hospitals. In the absence of a medieval bureaucracy engaged in the provision and supervision of relief, and given the dearth of comprehensive documentation relating to poverty and the poor, medieval hospitals seem to provide one of the few areas offering scope for a close study of the experience of poverty and its relief. Medieval hospitals were usually endowed institutions, and since they often existed under the tutelage of the church, they generated a variety of legal and ecclesiastical documentation. In the countryside, these institutions owned land and were involved in the business of parochial as well as manorial administration; in towns, they often acted in the urban property market, leaving their mark in sources related to the purchase and exchange of tenements, in rentals, and in records of ownership disputes. Through the careful juxtaposition of these materials it is possible to trace the institutional histories of individual hospitals, and occasionally, wherever statutes, rules, exceptional law-suits or evidence of benefactions have survived, we are allowed a glimpse into a hospital's day-to-day life. But these glimpses are rare and, on the whole, do *not* allow us to recreate a full picture of the nature of life, relief and patronage experienced in the medieval hospital. That this is so is a source of frustration to those of us who have studied hospitals as 'bridges' to the poor, as well as of exasperation to some of the readers of our works.[1]

But it is not the absence of material alone which blights the study of medieval hospitals and the poor treated in them. Those

14

reading descriptions of medieval hospitals often complain about the unfamiliar nature of such institutions: medieval hospitals seem to fulfil only a few of the functions expected of them by our contemporaries. No matter how good our archive we hear little of the type of medical care, the number of inmates and their ailments, little about rates of cure, regimes and routines maintained in these houses. Occasionally a stray kitchen account, a fragment of a work of art, a testament, or a tax-return, may provide a more detailed picture of hospital life, and these are triumphantly highlighted by the historian.[2] But through such flashes we seldom capture the sense of routine, of the nature of relief offered, of treatment, or of subsequent cure and recuperation, let alone a picture of the social relations which developed under and around the hospital's roof. To complicate matters, not only have medieval hospitals left very little evidence about treatment, but they additionally, and maddeningly, emerge as institutions in which a whole array of non-medical activities took place. They were venues for money-lending, liturgical practice and intercession, for pastoral work, a retirement-house for elderly and well-to-do burgesses, they could provide accommodation for clerics and students, and scope for speculation in the land-market. The discovery of such non-caring activities under the guise of charity has induced some critics to claim that medieval charitable activity was a myth, and that looking at hospitals is an ill-conceived project.[3] Such critics would maintain, and not without some reason, that far more effective, and far more revealing, are those studies which aim to explore forms of communal relief and mutual help which took place outside institutions and to a large extent informally, within family, in provision for the aged in rural communities, in neighbourly help, in other words, in the moral economy of pre-industrial society.

Such a 'structural' approach to arrangements for relief, which imputes to them a strong fit to other social institutions and which falls in with demographic and economic features, is undoubtedly true. Thus provision for need within a system where extended families prevailed will differ from that arising where nuclear families are the rule. Furthermore, the structure of rural indigence and of urban poverty, and even within these spheres the distinct types of 'shallow' and 'deep' poverty recently discussed by Paul Slack,[4] each requires different solutions and can be contained by differing preventives. And this has, on the whole, been ignored.

Yet no matter how diverse and structurally embedded the provisions for need, there is another area of concern which can hardly be ignored, and which is none the less ill-captured within models that attempt to fit the demand for, with the supply of, relief. Mediating between need and its relief are the processes of identification and interpretation of need, the decision to act, and the formulation of strategies for action in the minds of those able to relieve. This sphere is almost totally neglected by students of relief institutions, and it is particularly here that a fresh look at hospitals could now yield rich returns. In their shifting usages and meanings hospitals reflect changes in the choices and in the priorities of relief, they force us to consider the ways in which relief and social responsibility were perceived, and more importantly, how these were understood and constituted in a given culture. Relief is always a product of deliberation; and it is discursively constructed. Since we shall never recover the whole web of relations which constituted a 'moral economy' of the Middle Ages, we are in fact forced to contend with the dynamic interactions operating at the loci of charity, relief and exchange. As we do so, we shall uncover the *language* of relief, within which the predicted and structurally fitting solutions, their choice or their rejection, made sense, and without which or outside of which, they come to us bearing altogether little meaning.

To say this is to step away from any functionalist approach which would see straightforward and effective processes of adjustment determining responses to new social realities. Rather, to speak of a discourse of charity is not to talk of a single position on charity, nor of a necessary fit between it and some objective need experienced by the poor. It is rather to insist that 'objective' need is never transparently encountered by us or by our historical actors, but rather a version seen in terms of a discourse on social obligation, well-being, merit and virtue which interprets the problem and within which responses to it are constructed. And this response can fail or succeed in meeting experienced need, or in agreeing with other discourses on charity and poverty. The discourse of charity then problematizes and makes the indigence of others more or less relevant to those able to redistribute. Allocation of resources does not operate 'efficiently' since maintenance and relief of as many people as possible is not a coherent or a universal interest by any means, nor is it universally and similarly perceptible by all. Yet relief systems do evolve, a degree of redistribution is effected in most societies, and as such it is always negotiated within the domain where culture and politics merge, through the language of social relations and its attendant meanings. In other words, there is no reason to assume that an equilibrium between supply and demand for relief is an aim, even in cases where serial material allows us subtly to trace the creation of such a balance, without due consideration of the variety of aims which motivate charitable action. The relation between need and provision is mediated through a nexus of perceptions of social roles, of the nature of relations and obligations, of the symbolic value of giving and receiving. Furthermore, in deployment and use of the language of relief different understandings of responsibility can coexist: those of the laity and the clergy, of men and women, of merchants and artisans, burgesses and peasants. The boundaries of responsibility become more clearly articulated only when a system of subscription is enforced, and even then the meaning of contribution and the assessment of a system's adequacy cannot be gathered merely from formal pronouncements. Even when relief is bureaucratically provided, measured against allegedly universal standards, the ongoing nature of need and of the imperative which engages friends and strangers to relieve it, is constructed within a cultural field which we must identify and consider.

To acknowledge this is not to dispute the strong correlations between types of material need and the particular forms of provision designed to meet them. Indeed, the link is powerfully demonstrated in Richard Smith's analysis of the provision for aged tenants within the manorial system,[5] or in the types of distributions devised by Italian charities such as Or San Michele in fourteenth-century Florence.[6] But a *language* of charity and obligation interposes between the identification of need, its interpretation, and finally the response to it. This language articulates incentives to altruistic behaviour, but harbours a considerable variety of possible courses of action, so varied at times that it can provide avenues for evasion on the issue of giving, resulting in a less than efficient system. What is most striking in popular religious instruction of the later Middle Ages is just such broadness and variety of demands for charitable action, within a powerful idiom of charity and brotherhood.[7] Medieval hospitals existed within this cultural setting, and were designed and shaped by it; this is to say that involvement in their foundation or maintenance through benefaction was no simple response to normative religious dictates.

Looking at medieval hospitals and identifying the language of charity within which they were conceived need not imply a blindness on our part towards the power relations which this language legitimized, nor an acceptance on our part of the merits or necessity of any given language of charity, its virtue or its aptness. Rather, by looking at hospitals, at the variety of activities practised within them in the idiom of charity, one can explore the range of possible meanings existing within this language. By discerning the preference of particular meanings of charity over others, and through the effect of such choices on the fortunes of hospitals, we can learn some hard facts about attitudes which settle on one, rather than on another, of the meanings existing within the charitable array. Potential givers were constantly assessing the fit of their actions with their resources in terms of the charitable idiom, to produce the most satisfying package of social and spiritual reward. The language in which grants to hospitals were made was that also used to describe the terms of loans arranged between hospital and patron, or even to establish outright sales between them. The impulse towards engagement in the public action of endowment and benefaction was influenced by ideas about well-being and social responsibility, as well as by an acute analysis of the elements of order and harmony in the town. All these evaluations were determined by the scope of meanings which the attendant language of charity offered, by the images of virtue, of merit and of intent which it recognized. Inasmuch as this language of charity was effective, it had to mediate between different groups and interests and in late medieval towns, from which most of our know-ledge of medieval hospitals survives, between the clerical discourse and that of civic government and politics. Here in their ability to provide a variety of rewards, the hospitals fit into an ethos of exchange characteristic both of the current religious language and of urban culture. By looking at the charitable decisions made around hospitals one can discover a field of social interaction, through which much that is usually lost in purely institutional studies can be learnt. This reveals the symbolic values which lent acts of giving their meaning, and gave the giver his or her incentive to act, and more or less satisfaction.

Let me exemplify these possibilities through an urban hospital which I have studied closely, the hospital of St John the Evangelist in Cambridge, and against the background of many similar in-stitutions.[8] The hospital was founded early in the thirteenth century by a group of burgesses from the leading families of the borough. The Dunnings and Blangernons together with tens of more modest burgesses provided the initial endowment in the form of tenements in the hospital's vicinity, lucrative properties in and around the market-square, together with tens of acres in the Cambridge fields and in neighbouring villages. To some extent their initiative was innovative;

it was the product of the type of deliberation and sense of control and responsibility which burgesses were experiencing and expressing in the growing boroughs in the twelfth and thirteenth centuries. But the new venture in relief of sickness and poverty depended to a large extent on pre-existing models of organization. That is to say that choices and preferences formulated in the realm of urban politics and administration were being expressed through a prevalent language of charity, and poured into administrative forms borrowed from the religious sphere. This sphere provided early hospital founders with legal and organizational frameworks for perpetual endowment, for the enforcement of collective responsibility, for supervision and auditing, all within an idiom of charity with its attendant rewards. So the hospital was the product of a convergence of aims, capabilities and models and the inspiration of need, of utility and of virtue. The symbolic value of the charitable institution further allowed a whole host of activities to be pursued within its walls. That this is so cannot be adequately explained by recourse to a cynical claim that the patrons could do as they wished with their creature, because they could not. As a public venue, as a collective and communal institution, the hospital was watched and controlled, through the knowledge of its workings and perceptions about its tasks and merits. During the period which I have studied, three centuries of the central and later Middle Ages, reformulations redrew the lines between the groups involved in hospital foundation and management, and reorientated the understandings of responsibility through a complex process of observation and rationalization on the part of those who were able to provide relief. What I claim is that as the notions of shared enterprise and deserving need changed, the nature of activities within the public sphere, such as activities in and around hospitals, changed too. There are, of course, limits to the imaginable and practicable uses of a given institution, especially one which purported to serve the general weal, and which functioned by virtue of an idiom of charity, co-operation and responsibility. Thus the new activities maintained by medieval hospitals were not spurious; be they the maintenance of students, intercessory prayers or provision of sinecures, they reflect the scope of action legitimized and at least recognized by those controlling them. They are within the boundaries of the prevailing language of charity.

This is not to deny that some very simple determinants of a more material nature do influence the fortunes of houses of relief. The incidence of endemic disease, plagues, war, demographic trends, all

19

will affect the forms and scope of relief. The virtual disappearance of many small rural hospitals from our records in the second half of the fourteenth century attests to the fact that small hospitals either literally died out or, in the case of those whose income was derived chiefly from land, could no longer subsist on their much depleted incomes after the sharp fall in land values after 1350. Similarly the foundation of leper hospitals and their subsequent demise with the decline of leprosy reflects the influence of external factors. This is fairly obvious; what is being stressed here is the way in which less obvious factors influence the fortunes of relief institutions, and attention is being drawn to less tangible and thus usually neglected influences.

When the inhabitants of the growing boroughs of twelfth- and thirteenth-century England engaged in the foundation of a hospital, this undertaking was envisaged as a collective enterprise similar to their control of the market, their supervision of water and food supplies, their maintenance of security. Hospitals founded by groups of leading burgesses often occupied sites which had been provided by the commonalty, or which had been purchased by one of their number. In the act of foundation a maturity of the collective urban enterprise was demonstrated, and yet within this co-operative endeavour some distinctly personal aims were being achieved: in personal rewards in the form of commemoration, through involvement in the management of the hospital's property, in the facility of buying, selling and borrowing from a well-disposed institution, and finally through participation in acts laden with symbolic expressions of largesse, of authority, of virtue – of power. Even if we must go some way in agreeing with those who take cynical positions about the value of studying charitable institutions as indicators of aggregate levels of relief, or of attitudes directed at the poor, we cannot overlook or deny the value of such a study in revealing the relevant understandings which underlay any participation in the distribution of wealth. The type of relief and the ways in which they were linked to particular social and political objectives of the powerful provide perhaps the most interesting point of entry into the vast area of unwritten, informal and yet expected behaviours which we would all agree governed and produced a large part of relief opportunities. So a hospital's records usually fail to tell us about the number of the poor, about levels of deprivation, about treatment. They can, however, reveal some of the occasions on which the interests and choices of the 'haves' produced redistributive activities and sustained relief institutions for others.

An important principle guiding the choices of those undertaking charitable initiatives was that of comparison and analogy in organizational forms. What strikes one in the earliest institutional articulations of charitable impulses, is that they borrowed and tested forms which had developed in other spheres. The attempt to endow an institution perpetually, to protect it from intrusion and to create in it a continuous flow of charitable-liturgical practice was met, in the twelfth and thirteenth centuries, by adoption of organizational forms from the sphere of secular religious life. Hospitals followed the patterns of secular collegiate houses – largely encompassed within the Augustinian rule – as religious institutions which functioned separately and independently within the secular world, ones which were provided with tools for self-management, and with means of subsistence for a perpetual body of priests and servants. The collegiate form was an important creation of the central Middle Ages, providing an alternative to the traditional forms of religious life in retreat in monasteries in the countryside, and it suggested itself to laymen as an attractive framework for the creation of a repository of charitable funds. Within such units a group of clerics – administrators, chaplains, servants – and inmates could be perpetually maintained, and the endowment could be held and protected under the multitude of exemptions, privileges and safeguards which applied to ecclesiastical properties. That an organizational pattern which had developed in the religious sphere was adopted to service the communal experiment in relief in towns does *not* imply any primacy to the spiritual motivations behind such acts. It was a safe and sensible choice in the early years of borough organization, when notions of and instruments for corporate projects were yet in their infancy, and when ecclesiastical endowment had already evolved over hundreds of years.

In the nature of institutional foundations which are meant to enhance prestige, the personal symbolic act of giving was always of vital importance in the charitable exchange. In these undertakings there always seems to have been an initial enthusiasm generated by the moment of hospital foundation, the crucial stage of planting and supporting the seedling institution, when each contribution seemed to leave a greater mark on the house's well-being. This phase was usually followed by a decline in interest after a generation or two. As the hospital became an accepted and familiar part of the local topography, grand efforts of endowment were gradually diverted to other objects. It is also true that of the multitude of benefactors who supported an urban charity, only a minority made this grand type of endowing contribution; for most benefactors the contribution was small, a few shillings in annual rent, some strips in the fields outside town or in a neighbouring village, just enough to keep them within the enterprise. Thus many hospitals founded in the later twelfth and thirteenth centuries attracted patronage, albeit at a constantly depleting rate, for even a century later. But this institutional dynamic (with a shower of smaller donations after the first endowing thrust), which can be found in hospitals in different periods, is not insensitive to contextual circumstances. Endowment can occur in an atmosphere which is, on the whole, favourable to collective action, or in one which is not. The examination of the whole variety of charitable choices within a town or a region, the inquiry whether the fall off in *some* is countered by the setting up of *different* types of institutions, can teach us about clusters of shifting understandings and attitudes towards the charitable act.

So it is possible to discern meaningful changes in attitudes among those who are in a position to give, through their choice of new enterprises or their adherence to old ones. Throughout the thirteenth and early fourteenth centuries a certain continuity, albeit with declining frequency, is noticeable in the foundation and maintenance trends of charitable houses. But the later fourteenth century produced a dramatically altered picture. It is extremely difficult to date these shifts, and neatly to correlate them to the more rigorous and detailed picture which we now possess of demographic and economic change in the period. Yet it is absolutely clear that the foundation of hospitals was rarer in these decades, and that in the appropriate sources complaints about the corrupt nature of those institutions multiply, complaints about the changed nature of institutions which had survived from the phase of intensive foundation a century earlier. Here, interests and expectations of different groups in the town were clashing over the language of charity.

This development is reflected in evidence from hospital cartularies and endowment charters. In those cases where sequences of donation can be reconstructed from the late thirteenth and in the fourteenth century, donations were falling off in Cambridge. While arrangements for private chantry-services within the hospital increased in number, the mention of poor and sick folk gradually disappeared, the number of corrodians (those holding lifelong retirement pensions in the hospital) multiplied – before our very eyes the hospital passes through stages of perception and construction. It survived through change. New types of charity and – in Cambridge – the provision of services for scholars were practised within its walls.

In parallel to this process of reinterpretation of the activities and of the services provided in and expected from a hospital we can also discern a clear trend among burgesses, gentry and substantial tenants in the countryside to engage in other types of charitable enterprises. This can be called a sectional trend, one which is reflected in choices of more narrowly defined groups as the venues for social, charitable or religious action. These could be an age-group, an occupational group, a parish, a village or a fraternity. In fraternities the adoption of fictive kinship underpins the provision of a whole range of social services within this closely knit group: funerary services, prayers for the dead, dowering of daughters, visiting the sick, relief of dependants. But the horizon of such mutual help was none the less a narrow one: late medieval parishes, guilds and fraternities took good care, but only of their own.

The adoption of more restricted frameworks of social action reflects changes in the understanding of the nature of obligation and co-operation within society: areas in which charity was practised acquired new meanings, their imperatives guided to different paths of action. Even within existing institutions the charitable balance was being dramatically transformed in the later Middle Ages. And these changes can be characterized as a tendency to privilege those who are familiar and similar, in the replication of uniformities of interest, outlook and potential need in the new forms of charitable organization. Moved by such considerations people were choosing partners and recipients in social action more *like* themselves, rather than engaging in visions of transformation of society through the general contribution towards the alleviation of need and distress. This is charity between similars, not others. Although the language of medieval Christian charity always required a degree of help to 'others', a different and alternative idiom, an idiom of kinship, spiced with some of the traditional images of charity and love, came to articulate new choices. This development can be correlated to similar manifestations of the nature of co-operation in the structures of late medieval town government, in the preponderance of faction within it, and in the more tentative attitudes towards public office by those who would have constituted the natural office-holding elite in earlier times.[9] It is also strongly related to the perceived reality of a generally higher standard of living among workers and, inasmuch as the profits of master-craftsmen and landowners alike were declining, a lesser ability of those better off to allocate charitable funds. Consequent to all these trends, charity was becoming more discriminating and discrete in a period when it was arguably less acutely needed, yet needed still.

These shifts in the language of charity, in which the dispositions towards giving were enshrined, were thoroughgoing and dramatic. The symbolic articulation of the charitable act was being wrested from its earlier institutional forms which were relatively open and inclusive; these older forms were being redesigned to ensure greater exclusivity and discrimination in allocation of relief funds, and altogether new types of relief were created in substantially altered social contexts.[10]

The hospital, then, was constructed and reconstructed within the changing language of charity through which social relations were experienced and explored. From a locus in which the reaches of co-operation and initiatives towards collective religious and social action could be explored in the twelfth and thirteenth centuries, it became the place where social pathologies (begging, prostitution, leprosy, venereal disease, as well as the unavoidable old age) were treated. And the more relaxed and generous-minded sharing and distribution was taking place in formations which brought together not complementary needs, but similar and familiar friends who helped each other. In addition these groups supervised not only almshouses that they might enter but also those remaining administrative charges: the surviving urban hospitals.

Through the study of such charitable/uncharitable institutions we discern attitudes which necessarily influenced the fabric of relations between groups and individuals at work-places, in families, in neighbourhoods. They would have shaped responses to requests for doorstep relief, the disposition towards provision of short-term loans, of help in time of crisis. Hospitals existed between need, the disposition to acknowledge need and the perceived responsibility to alleviate need; their history is sensitive to the interplay of these forces. They are venues wrought by the language of charity and in which this language's mandates and licences were explored. If the poor often fail to emerge as free agents in this type of historical tale it is because in many ways they were not free to act in this field. They were perceived and imagined – and inasmuch as they impinged on the consciousness of abler strangers, patrons and neighbours – charitable houses were imagined for their relief.

NOTES

1 See P. Horden, 'A discipline of relevance: the historiography of the later medieval hospital', *Social History of Medicine*, 1988, vol. 1, a review article of a number of studies of hospitals, including M. Rubin, *Charity and Community in Medieval Cambridge*, Cambridge, 1987.

2 See for example Harvey Dunning's donation of bedding for the Hospital of St John, Cambridge, and the kitchen accounts thereof: Rubin, op. cit., p. 161.

3 See C. Dyer's review in *Social History*, 1988, vol. 13.

4 P. Slack, *Poverty and Policy in Tudor and Stuart England*, London, 1988.

5 R. M. Smith, 'The manorial court and the elderly tenant in England 1250–1500', in Z. Razi and R. M. Smith (eds) *Manorial Court and Medieval Rural Society*, Oxford, forthcoming 1992.

6 J. S. Henderson, *Piety and Charity in Late Medieval Florence*, forthcoming 1992, chs 7 and 8.

7 See Rubin, op. cit., ch. 3.

8 See ibid., chs 4 and 5, and the comparative bibliography there.

9 See for example R. H. Britnell, *Growth and Decline in Colchester 1300–1525*, Cambridge, 1986; C. Phythian-Adams, *Desolation of a City: Coventry and the Urban Crisis of the Late Middle Ages*, Cambridge, 1979.

10 On some of these developments see M. Rubin, 'Development and change in English hospitals, 1100–1500', in L. Granshaw and R. Porter (eds) *The Hospital in History*, London, 1989, especially pp. 53–6.

2

HEALING THE POOR

Hospitals and medical assistance in Renaissance Florence

Katharine Park

Describing the city of Florence in 1527, the chronicler Benedetto Varchi divided its hospitals into two main groups: those that provided food and lodging for the healthy and those that (in Varchi's words) 'take in the sick' and 'supply them with medical care until they are well'. The first group embraced a miscellany of homes for widows and foundlings, hostels for travellers and pilgrims, and other smaller institutions, of which few, according to Varchi, 'function as they should, partly because their directors cannot see to it, and partly because they will not'. The second group, the hospitals for the sick, which Varchi described with evident and contrasting pride, included five large institutions, of which the principal was Santa Maria Nuova, with its awesome annual budget of 25,000 scudi.[1]

Varchi's admiring account of Florence's hospitals for the sick, which was echoed by many other writers of the fifteenth and sixteenth centuries, flies in the face of the common assumption that the hospital as we know it, devoted to offering professionally supervised medical care to sick people, developed only much later. Historians of medicine, ever anxious to isolate modern medicine from its benighted past, used to locate the emergence of this kind of hospital in the years around 1900; more recent writers have pushed it back to the late eighteenth, or even into the seventeenth century.[2] Despite such differences, however, most historians continue to assume that before this period professional medical care – such as it was – was a luxury enjoyed only by the urban elites, while the sick poor made do with home nursing, traditional healers and, as a last resort, the general spiritual, moral and custodial (but not medical) services that hospitals offered them together with many other groups of dependent souls.

26

As a number of recent studies have suggested, this interpretation demands revision. We are beginning to learn about the sophisticated medical hospitals that flourished in the cities of the medieval Islamic world as well as their smaller and paler Byzantine shadows.[3] Word of these eastern institutions made its way to western Europe as early as the late twelfth century, probably through the crusading order of the Hospitallers, or Knights of St John, and although the importance of eastern influence is still unclear, there was also a significant medical element in late medieval French hospitals.[4] The case is even stronger for Italy, where city life was much more developed, and where thriving urban economies could support a level of charity unknown elsewhere in Europe. In late medieval and Renaissance Italy, as in the Byzantine and Islamic east, hospitals for the sick were charitable organizations. Founded and funded by private individuals, religious orders, guilds, confraternities, and municipal and state governments, they formed part of an extensive network of public and private institutions designed to provide professional medical care to the population of city and countryside, with special attention to the needs of the poor.

The fourteenth and fifteenth centuries were pivotal in the emergence of hospitals for the sick and other forms of medical assistance. During this period, Italian lay piety moved away from traditional ascetic forms towards a concern with social problems that engaged the whole community.[5] Contemporaries understood well the reciprocal links between poverty and disease. Poverty bred disease, and vice versa: the illness or death of a wage-earner could catapult his or her family into the ranks of the indigent. Furthermore, Christian scripture and tradition identified the sick as particularly deserving of charity. Thus from 1300 on, the 'sick poor', as they were known, appeared with increasing frequency alongside widows, foundlings, travellers, the aged, and disabled people as a special group with a recognized claim to social assistance.[6]

The problem of the sick poor gained a special urgency from the middle of the fourteenth century on, as a series of epidemics swept through the overpopulated Italian cities. The most fearful of these diseases was plague. City-dwellers quickly identified plague with the poor; during the Black Death of 1348, according to the Florentine chronicler Matteo Villani, 'the lower and middle orders suffered more than the upper classes, because they were weaker to begin with, because they were hit first and hardest, and because they had less help and lived in worse conditions'.[7] As Villani recorded, these epidemics produced a flood of charitable bequests and foundations. They also focused public and private attention on the problem of providing medical care for the poor. This concern sprang from several distinct but mutually reinforcing considerations. Citizens wished to alleviate the suffering of the sick, both out of genuine concern for the poor and out of fear that the recurrent epidemics represented God's punishment for their own lack of charity, among other sins.[8] Employers and officials worried about the dramatic depopulation of Italian cities, the scarcity of labour and the resultant rise in wages; in addition to encouraging immigration by grants of citizenship and other privileges, they had good reason to invest in the health and productivity of their workers.[9] They also hoped to prevent and contain the spread of epidemic disease in the cities by attending to the fragile health of the poor, whom they saw as a perpetual reservoir of potential infection, and by providing places for them to be treated and isolated when the presence of plague was confirmed.[10]

The proposed solutions to these problems varied from city to city, even within the relatively homogeneous world of northern and central Italy, and changed significantly over time, as governments and individuals learned from experience and altered their understanding of disease and their religious, social, political and economic priorities. For this reason, local studies are crucial. We cannot, for example, take the coercive social hygiene of the fifteenth-century duchy of Milan as typical of the much more decentralized world of the Venetian and Florentine republics, and we should not project backward the harsher attitudes toward poverty that began to appear in the early sixteenth century.[11] During the earlier period, Venice invested heavily in communal doctors, while Milan and the Lombard towns developed public health measures controlling the movements of infected or potentially infected groups.[12] But perhaps the most important product of this period of experimentation for the history of health care – and certainly the most famous offspring of the marriage of charity and medicine – was the large hospital for the sick poor, designed to mobilize all the resources of contemporary medicine to cure its patients and to allow them quickly to resume their regular life and work. Tuscany in general, and Florence in particular, were at the forefront of this development; their specialized medical hospitals, particularly the great Florentine hospital of Santa Maria Nuova, became models to be admired, if not copied, in other Italian cities and eventually throughout Europe.[13]

My aim in this chapter is to give an account of medical organization and practice in the four great Florentine hospitals for the sick in the fourteenth and fifteenth centuries, concentrating on Santa Maria Nuova and, to a lesser extent, San Paolo. (The fifth hospital mentioned by Varchi, Santissima Trinità of the Incurables, founded in 1520, was, I shall argue, a somewhat different institution.) I hope to show that by the early sixteenth century these hospitals had as their principal function the primary care of the acutely ill and that they had subsumed many of the functions of the earlier Florentine institutions, notably public surgeons and charitable associations, that concerned themselves with the sick poor. They had developed a set of specialized administrative procedures that allowed them to provide individualized therapy to large numbers of patients, and they had begun to establish a special relationship to the medical profession, providing formal and informal training for medical students and recently graduated physicians in exchange for professional services. They were in this sense clearly medical institutions; at the same time, the medical care they offered conformed to their conception of medicine rather than ours and must be understood in that context.

Although the hospital for the sick became the principal vehicle for providing free medical care to the poor, it was neither the earliest nor initially the most important such institution. Florence, unlike cities such as Parma and Urbino, did not require its doctors to treat the poor without charge, but local practitioners had long done so as private acts of piety and charity.[14] By the early fourteenth century, however, it had become clear that such casual and incidental assistance could not meet the medical needs of the growing number of Florentine indigents, prompting the commune to hire its first public doctor.

The institution of the public doctor, first documented in the early thirteenth century, was by that time well established in Italy; in 1324, for example, Venice paid salaries to thirteen physicians and eighteen surgeons, whose income from private practice was supplemented in return for free treatment of the poor.[15] Florence chose to adopt a more economical and less comprehensive model, which consisted of supporting a much smaller number of doctors to provide specialized medical treatment to a particular group of poor patients, those who required straightforward surgical operations. In 1326 it hired Iacopo dell'Ossa of Rome – a specialist in fractures and dislocations, as his name implied – to treat without charge 'the people of the city and countryside of Florence, . . . particularly those without resources [impotentes] and the poor'. Initially granted only a small salary and an allowance to maintain his horse, he soon received a highly unusual tax exemption, later guaranteed by city statute to all public 'bone doctors'.[16] The city gradually expanded its roster of public doctors over the next forty years – and notably after the Black Death in 1348 – employing by 1361 a total of five: two bone doctors; a doctor to prisoners and condemned criminals; an eye doctor; and a man specializing in the treatment of 'eyes, hernias, boils, fractures, and dislocations'.[17] Their ranks shrank rapidly from that year on, leaving only the prison doctor on the public payroll after 1370.

Even at its height, however, the medical care offered by Florence's public doctors was limited in scope. All belonged to a particular group within the medical profession: empirical surgeons skilled in a particular operation or group of operations – setting fractures, rectifying dislocations, lancing and dressing boils, treating hernias, and couching cataracts.[18] They specialized, in other words, in diseases which were extremely common, acute but rarely life-threatening, and highly treatable within the framework of contemporary medical knowledge. They could put able-bodied workers back on their feet, but did not attend those suffering from internal illnesses requiring closer supervision and longer-term treatment. This strategy was not peculiar to Florence – Milan and many other smaller towns chose to invest their resources in this way[19] – and it clearly represented a highly specific and cost-effective investment in the health of its labouring class.

The commune's narrow approach to providing medical care for the poor may also have reflected the view that those who needed the services of a physician rather than a surgeon had other forms of recourse. If they were neither too sick nor too poor, they could repair to one of Florence's many pharmacies, where physicians employed by the shopkeeper held regular clinics, and patients had to pay only for the medicines prescribed. Or, if they could afford the annual dues, they could join one of the religious confraternities that by the middle of the fifteenth century were beginning to provide their members with physicians, together with other social services such as dowries and burials.[20] Those too poor to pay for either of these alternatives were thrown back on private or corporate charity. The great charitable company of Or San Michele occasionally sent doctors to their homes,[21] local physicians might offer their services, or the fee might be paid by a neighbour or other member of the formal and informal networks of assistance that operated in the Florentine neighbourhoods and parishes.[22] The principal resort of the sick poor from the middle of the fourteenth century on, however, was undoubtedly the city's hospitals.

Of the roughly thirty-five hospitals active in Florence in the later fourteenth and fifteenth centuries, most were not organized to provide specialized medical care for the sick. They were rather general charitable institutions established and supported by private citizens, guilds and confraternities to offer short- or long-term shelter and maintenance to the needy, variously defined.[23] Some were reserved for the members of a particular trade, such as the hospital of San Giovanni Decollato, founded in 1317 for old, sick, and poor porters, or the slightly later hospitals of Sant'Onofrio, for dyers, and Santissima Trinità, for shoemakers. Several – notably, from the middle of the fifteenth century on, Santa Maria degli Innocenti – took in foundlings, while others served pilgrims and travellers or 'poor women' or simply 'the poor'. Most were very small institutions, the main exceptions being the three large foundling hospitals (San Gallo, Santa Maria della Scala, the Innocenti) and the Orbatello, a home for poor women; few of the others had more than eight or ten beds, and some had only two or three.[24]

It is difficult to find detailed information about the people taken in by these hospitals, but the evidence suggests that, with the exception of the hospitals for children and travellers, many of their beds were occupied by the old and chronically ill. Thus the seven women residents of the hospital of the Divote della Vergine Maria in 1428, for example, included a 60-year-old widow, 'blind and sick'; an 80-year-old widow, 'sick and doesn't get out of bed'; a 50-year-old, 'tired out and sick'; and a 25-year-old woman, who 'has been sick for more than a year with an illness from which she will not recover until she dies'.[25] Two other small hospitals, San Iacopo a Sant'Eusebio, the leprosarium, and Sant'Antonio, for those infected or crippled by the disease or diseases known as Saint Anthony's Fire, were devoted exclusively to incurably ill and disabled people.[26] Except for the foundling hospitals, none of these had doctors on their regular payrolls, and there is no evidence to suggest that they were organized to offer their sick residents more than basic nursing and shelter. In this they differed profoundly from the great Florentine hospitals for the sick poor.

By 1400 there were four of these latter institutions in the city: Santa Maria Nuova (founded in 1289); San Paolo (thirteenth century); San Giovanni, also called 'di messer Bonifazio' after the mercenary captain who established it (1377); and San Matteo, also called 'di

Lemmo' (1389).[27] The last two were founded as general hospices and began to limit their attention to the sick in the third and fourth decades of the fourteenth century, while the latter two were established exclusively for that purpose. All were relatively large institutions: the last three had places for between fifty and seventy-five patients, while Santa Maria Nuova normally housed between two and three hundred. Unlike the leprosarium, they were not places for isolating or warehousing the sick; all four paid salaries to a professional medical staff that included physicians, surgeons and pharmacists. Santa Maria Nuova, for example, employed two (male) doctors in the fourteenth century, three in the early fifteenth, four in 1450, and ten in 1500. By 1376 it had a fully equipped pharmacy on the premises.[28] The doctors were assisted by a resident staff of laymen (*servi*) or laywomen (*servae*), who had donated their possessions to the hospital, taking a vow of obedience and assuming the hospital's grey habit with its emblem of a red and green crutch. Both men and women acted as nurses in their respective wards, while the women also attended to the monumental task of cooking, cleaning and laundering for the hospital's hundreds of dependants. In addition, several women – probably drawn from among the *servae* – were described as doctors (*medicae*).[29]

The dramatic rise in the number of doctors employed by Santa Maria Nuova over the fourteenth and fifteenth centuries reflects less an increase in the number of its patients, which seems to have remained generally stable, than an elaboration of the medical services it offered. We can appreciate this change by comparing two documents: the hospital statute from 1374 and the statute sent to Henry VII of England shortly after 1500.[30] Although it referred to medical treatment in the hospital, the former concentrated on religious and moral prescriptions – sacraments, religious offices, duties of the priests, restrictions on male visits to the women's part of the hospital, and so forth. The latter, on the other hand, while still emphasizing these aspects of the hospital, also reveals a fully formed and highly developed system of health care. It describes the hospital as divided into two main wards, for men and women. The male ward alone housed a hundred double beds made up with mattresses, bolsters, pillows, linens and covers, and numbered to identify individual patients. The hospital employed a full-time pharmacist, with four apprentices, as well as a staff of ten doctors. The three most junior lived and worked in the hospital in return for room, board and clinical experience. They were supervised by six senior physicians, described as 'the most illustrious in the entire city', who came every morning to examine the sick, listen to the reports of the nurses, and issue prescriptions for the care of each patient. Special classes of patients – including the mentally ill 'from physical causes', those with head wounds, and those with skin lesions – were isolated from the general wards and from each other. The last two groups were treated by a seventh senior doctor, a surgeon, who came to the hospital for two hours each morning and evening.[31]

As the statute makes clear, the patients in Santa Maria Nuova, except when brought unconscious to the hospital, presented themselves voluntarily for admission and were discharged in the same way. During their stay in hospital they received free medical care in the form of food, drink and medications prepared especially for them and identified by the omnipresent bed number. Furthermore, the hospital not only served the poor, although this was its primary mission, but also received sick pilgrims, as well as patients of higher status who could not be cared for at home, either because they were travelling or because they had chosen to enter the hospital as part of a religious vow. (Popes Martin V and Sixtus IV had granted generous indulgence to all who served or died in the hospital.)[32] These patients were lodged in eight individual bedrooms with a fireplace, toilet and sink.

Finally, the hospital provided various medical services to the city at large. From the late fourteenth century on, it had acted as a medical lending library, supplying local surgeons and physicians with books in both Latin and Italian,[33] and as a public dispensary. Its front portico accommodated two great jars containing barley water for public use and the famous concentrated chicken broth with which it plied its patients; it supplied medical advice and vast quantities of medicines and medicated bandages to the city at large and to special groups such as prisoners in the city jail. It also provided surgical treatment to out-patients from the city and countryside suffering from 'sores and other minor illnesses' and sent out trained nurses into the city to treat seriously ill people at home.[34] In 1448 the commune appointed it to supervise the projected municipal plague hospital, San Bastiano.[35]

In this way, Santa Maria Nuova increasingly functioned as a general medical resource for the entire Florentine community, defining its primary mission in specifically medical terms. In other words, whereas it had been founded to serve the poor, with special emphasis on the sick, by the early sixteenth century it was serving the sick, with special emphasis on the poor. In pursuit of this mission, it had developed close ties with the organized and licensed medical profession in Florence. The care it offered was supervised by physicians and surgeons drawn from the city's elite. Over the course of the fifteenth century, for example, the 'house doctors', as they were called, included Fruosino di Cino Della Fioraia, many times consul of the Guild of Doctors, Apothecaries and Grocers; Piero di maestro Domenico dal Pozzo Toscanelli, richest physician in the city and brother of the humanist and scientist Paolo Toscanelli; Agostino di Stefano Santucci, professor of medicine at the University of Florence and later the occupant of a handsome tomb in the centre aisle of the church of Santa Croce; and Mariotto di Niccolò da Castiglione Aretino, the personal physician of Piero de' Medici.[36] Furthermore, by the middle of the sixteenth century, the medical profession itself was beginning to use the hospital as a centre for medical training; the College of Doctors recommended that graduates in medicine from the universities of Pisa and Siena practise in the hospital before attempting their licensing examination and required those who failed to extend their clinical training. By the beginning of the seventeenth century, Santa Maria Nuova housed a full-fledged school of surgery, later expanded to include formal training in lithotomy, ophthalmology, and medical botany and pharmacy.[37]

Like Santa Maria Nuova, the other three Florentine hospitals for the sick poor also developed over the course of the later fourteenth and fifteenth centuries a specialized medical organization that relied on the services of the medical profession. Just as important, they were apparently very selective in the patients they admitted, as is clear from the 'books of the sick' and the 'books of the dead' that survive in the archives of the hospitals of San Paolo and Santa Maria Nuova; these remarkable documents contain detailed information concerning hospital patients from the late fifteenth century on, including names, dates of admission and death or discharge, admission and bed numbers (in the case of male patients), and occasionally ages, occupations and diagnoses. These data reveal a striking and consistent pattern.[38] First, they testify to an unexpectedly low mortality. Over the decade between 1503 and 1512, for example, the average death-rate in Santa Maria Nuova was 10.5 per cent of the several thousand male patients received each year, and between 1518 and 1522 it averaged only 8.6 per cent.[39] The record of the much smaller hospital of San Paolo, which had only fifteen beds in its male ward and admitted several hundred men a year, was even better: from 1554 to 1561 an average of only 5.2 per cent of its male patients died in hospital; the rest received the annotation '*andòsene*' ('he went away').[40] Furthermore, the length of stay of the average male patient was unexpectedly short: about eight days for those who died in San Paolo and ten for those who left, and twenty-one days for those who died in Santa Maria Nuova. Among the dead males in both hospitals (and the sick in San Paolo), the great majority had been there twenty days or fewer.[41]

These figures raise as many questions as they answer. Not all of the discharged patients can be regarded as cured; some were doubtless only improved or left the hospital for other reasons.[42] None the less, the figures suggest that these hospitals functioned largely or exclusively as hospitals for the acutely rather than the chronically ill, and that the latter were excluded in the course of the diagnostic examination that according to the statutes preceded each admission. (There is no evidence that Santa Maria Nuova discharged chronically ill patients, once admitted; as we shall see, the case is less clear for syphilitics at San Paolo, who were occasionally sent either temporarily or permanently to the Incurabili.) This does not mean that the hospital accepted only mild or curable cases. The books of the dead contain many references to patients who were carried in without signs of life ('*non favilla*' and '*ben'è morta*' are common entries), expired under examination before even being assigned to a bed, or died during their first day in hospital. But it does imply that hospital administrators had made a conscious decision to concentrate their beds and their resources on patients who could be expected to die or recover in short order, making room for yet other sick poor.

This hypothesis is confirmed by what information we possess about the patients' illnesses. These were rarely noted in admissions and death records, with the exception of a single year, 1567–8, in which the infirmarer of San Paolo recorded diagnoses for nearly all the male patients admitted to his ward. During that time, the majority (220 out of almost 400 for whom diagnoses survive) had fevers of various sorts, 'fever' being a common term for a number of acute infections. The next largest group (about sixty patients) complained of skin diseases, ulcers and boils. A further twenty-three were admitted for accidental injuries, wounds, fractures and bites, while at least fifteen suffered from syphilis. The illnesses of the rest were miscellaneous, including haemorrhoids, exhaustion, cataracts, dysentery, smallpox, typhus and constipation.[43] Only very infrequently did the infirmarer indicate chronic conditions, such as phthisis, old age and dropsy; the sole exception was syphilis, which manifested itself in acute episodes. It is of course difficult to interpret these diagnostic categories and to identify in our terms the diseases to which they refer. It seems clear, however, that the vast majority of patients admitted to San Paolo in the mid-sixteenth century suffered from acute diseases or conditions.

The policy seems to have been somewhat different for female patients, as far as it is possible to judge from the erratic and rudimentary women's records of Santa Maria Nuova. The female ward had seventy beds, compared to the hundred in the male ward. Correspondingly fewer women seem to have been admitted, and their death-rate appears to have been somewhat higher.[44] Furthermore, the women who died in the hospital seem to have had a longer average length of stay – fifty-three days in 1518–19, as opposed to twenty-one for the men – and although the majority of them, like the men, left quickly, a significantly greater proportion stayed for periods of several months or, in a few cases, several years.[45] This suggests that the women's ward was far more crowded than the men's,[46] and that the women's hospital may have had a somewhat different policy concerning admissions. Women were disproportionately represented among the city's aged; the municipal books of the dead record twice as many women dying of old age as men.[47] The plight of Florence's many poor widows, together with the general Florentine fixation on women as particularly deserving objects of charity – the same combination of factors that combined to produce the Orbatello[48] – may have pressed the female wards to loosen their admissions criteria and to receive a larger number of women who were old, disabled or chronically ill.

None the less, the figures for both men and women in general belie the notion that all early hospitals were warehouses for old and terminally ill people or focuses of unchecked infection, places from which few returned alive; as the records show, people entered them voluntarily, expecting to get better, and their expectations were usually fulfilled. The effectiveness of the hospitals for the sick arose in large part from their admissions procedures, but it also reflected the nature of their therapeutics. Many acute illnesses are self-limiting and respond well to warmth, rest, nourishing food and simple surgical procedures. These were in fact the treatments of choice in this period, inside the hospitals and outside them. The distinction between care and cure did not exist in Renaissance medicine. Physicians shunned aggressive intervention, which they saw as dangerous to both patient and professional reputation, opting instead for conservative and supportive therapy. Contemporary medical writers often cited Galen's dictum, *Omnium natura operatrix, medicus vero minister*, to emphasize that the doctor's main task was to keep the patient alive and comfortable, strengthening the vital forces while the natural healing processes took their course: 'the art [of medicine]', as Niccolò Falcucci put it, 'is the image of nature and her follower'.[49] Thus physicians preferred to work through what they called 'regimen' or 'diet' – changes in food and drink, sleep, exercise, and so forth – although they recognized that medication was often necessary.[50] But even their drugs were extremely mild, composed for the most part of common herbal ingredients. Thus the sick were rarely subjected to the brutal measures, such as heroic bleeding and purging, that we wrongly associate with medicine in this period. Renaissance surgeons operated only as a last resort and even then, given the lack of anaesthesia or antisepsis, rarely opened the body cavity. They set fractures, fixed dislocations, bound or sutured wounds, and dressed sores and rashes – simple and effective operations that required little theoretical knowledge and lay well within their technical competence.

The description of Santa Maria Nuova for Henry VII confirms this picture, revealing an overriding concern with heating, food and drink (with an emphasis on concentrated chicken broth), and cleanliness. The hospital's account books echo this approach, with their massive expenditures on charcoal, linens, ashes (for laundry), and food as well as their meticulously kept lists of pharmaceutical supplies, ranging from common plant products to water imported from distant spas, to exorbitantly expensive items such as opium and gold leaf. The most detailed information on the medicines used in the Florentine hospitals for the sick comes from a voluminous notebook of medical recipes 'tried and tested in the hospital of Santa Maria Nuova'. The manuscript, compiled in 1515, includes preparations for a wide range of illnesses, from head wounds and arthritis to incontinence, irregular menstruation, insomnia, diarrhoea and worms. All were entirely naturalistic, made using mild, often herbal ingredients such as rosewater, wine, mustard, nettle seed, mastic, sugar, camphor, sandalwood, fennel and camomile. Many were attributed to the various 'house doctors' (including two women) associated with the hospital in the mid- to late fifteenth century, or borrowed from Michele di Mariano, the doctor at San Paolo. Some were evidently customized creations by particular doctors for particular patients:

Maestro Ficino's ointment 'for Dorotea's eye', for example, or the prescription 'for a woman whose mouth was filled with cankers, according to the recipe of Maestro Fruosino'.[51] Records of this sort confirm that hospital doctors and administrators aimed to provide individualized treatment to each patient and that they frequently exchanged or invented new recipes to that end.

As all these records imply, Florence's hospitals for the sick poor were organized and run primarily as therapeutic institutions for acutely ill people, taking the word 'therapeutic' to reflect the medical learning of the time. They were clearly differentiated from other, custodial hospitals, and they did not practise the 'medicine of confinement' that some historians, drawing on Lombard models and later practices, have assumed to be universal in fourteenth- and fifteenth-century Italy.[52] This becomes particularly clear if we consider the three principal diseases seen by contemporaries as contagious and therefore candidates for confinement and isolation: leprosy, plague and syphilis. The Florentine hospitals for the sick had never admitted lepers, who had their own institution as early as the twelfth century and who by the fifteenth century were too few to be of public concern. During the first century after 1348, they accepted plague victims, but this policy changed as plague came increasingly to be seen and managed as a contagious disease and a matter for public policing and control. By the mid-fifteenth century it was Florentine policy to put all plague victims in Santa Maria Nuova, thus isolating them from the sick poor in the other hospitals. This measure had obvious drawbacks, however, and as early as 1448 the city government developed plans for a special plague hospital that would remove plague victims from the regular hospitals entirely. In 1479 they were placed in the hospital of Santa Maria della Scala, previously occupied by foundlings but rendered obsolete by the new institution of the Innocenti, and in the years after 1500 they were removed outside the city walls to the new plague hospital of San Bastiano (staffed by its own medical personnel), the convent of San Salvi, and a shanty town of huts constructed especially for the purpose in the 1520s.[53] It was assumed, in other words, that the hospitals for the sick poor served a fundamentally different purpose from the *lazarettos* and other institutions for isolating contagiously ill patients.

Syphilis, which reached Florence in 1496, represented a different case. Seen, like plague, as contagious and associated to some extent with the poor, it moved some Italian cities to early exercises in coercive social hygiene.[54] Others, like Florence, chose to deal with the disease in another way. In 1520 a group of Florentine laymen and laywomen founded a special hospital, Santissima Trinità (called 'degli Incurabili') to receive syphilitics and other chronically ill poor. The new Florentine hospital for incurables did not function as an institution for isolation and confinement, like the plague hospital, but as the counterpart and complement to the hospitals for acutely ill people. As the statute of 1574 makes clear, even after the hospital had evolved into a specialized institution for syphilitics, which had not been the case in earlier decades, entrance was voluntary, and the burden was on the patient seeking admission to prove his or her eligibility – that he or she was both suffering from syphilis and poor.[55] And from the very beginning, Santissima Trinità conformed to the medical model developed in Santa Maria Nuova and other hospitals for the acutely ill poor; it hired doctors and surgeons, experimented with various forms of therapy (ultimately opting for treatment with guaiac wood), and quickly became a centre for medical research and teaching as well as practice. This appears clearly in the mid-sixteenth-century records of the hospital of San Paolo, which sent a number of its patients, syphilitics and others, to the Incurabili for the 'wood treatment', readmitting them to convalesce when their regimen of sweating, purging and drying was complete.[56]

In Renaissance Florence, therefore, the sick poor were not in general targets for isolation and confinement, except to some extent in the special case of plague, and the public and private forms of medical assistance available to them did not have that end in mind. There is no evidence that the communal surgeon acted as an agent of state surveillance, as one historian has argued, or the hospital for the sick as an instrument of 'repression' or 'segregation'.[57] In addition to being genuine expressions of Christian charity, these institutions were certainly tools of social policy, but the problem they aimed to solve was the chronic shortage of labour and rise in wages caused by recurrent epidemics of plague. Their principal intention, visible in clearest form in the choice of public doctors, was to offer free medical treatment of the highest quality possible to a well-defined sub-group of the Florentine poor: productive workers suffering from acute and treatable illnesses such as fractures, eye infections, hernias, fevers and skin diseases. Their goal, far from being one of confinement, was to cure these workers and return them to the labour force in the shortest time possible – a goal doubtless shared by the patients themselves.

The 1520s and 1530s saw a hardening of attitudes toward the poor and a concomitant change in the administration of poor relief in Florence as elsewhere in Italy.[58] By this time, however, the internal development of the Florentine hospitals for the sick poor was already largely complete, the result of two hundred years of evolution. This evolution took place on the level of social and institutional organization rather than intellectual system. The period in question saw no significant shifts in medical theory or therapeutics, no epistemic rupture in methodology or technique. We see instead the slow growth of a sense of civil interest in the health of the poor and a gradual but decisive development of specialized institutions to that end. These processes were accelerated during the fourteenth and fifteenth centuries by the prolonged medical and demographic crisis of plague, but not created by it. They form part of a communal flowering of medical institutions and medical organization visible in northern Italy well before 1348. And while the general system of poor relief was reorganized in the mid-sixteenth century, its constituent parts, including the large hospitals for the acutely ill poor, continued to develop in directions already well established during the late Middle Ages and Renaissance.

NOTES

1 B. Varchi, *Storia fiorentina*, ed. M. Santorio, 2 vols, Milan, 1845–6, vol. 1, p. 394.
2 For the older view, see for example H. E. Sigerist, 'An outline of the development of the hospital', *Bulletin of the History of Medicine*, 1936, vol. 4. Cf. M. Foucault, *The Birth of the Clinic: An Archeology of Medical Perception*, tr. A. M. Sheridan Smith, New York, 1975, esp. the introduction and chs 1 and 5; G. B. Risse, *Hospital Life in Enlightenment Scotland: Care and Teaching at the Royal Infirmary of Edinburgh*, Cambridge, 1986, e.g. p. 278.
3 For example M. Dols, 'The origins of the Islamic hospital: myth and reality', *Bulletin of the History of Medicine*, 1987, vol. 16; S. Hamarneh, 'Development of hospitals in Islam', *Journal of the History of Medicine and Allied Sciences*, 1962, vol. 17; T. S. Miller, *The Birth of the Hospital in the Byzantine Empire*, Baltimore, Md, 1985.
4 T. S. Miller, 'The Knights of Saint John and the hospitals of the Italian West', *Speculum*, 1978, vol. 53; M. Mollat, 'La vie quotidienne dans les hôpitaux médiévaux', in J. Imbert (ed.) *Histoire des hôpitaux en France*, Toulouse, 1982, pp. 130–3; E. Wickersheimer, 'Médecins et chirurgiens dans les hôpitaux du Moyen Age', *Janus*, 1928, vol. 32.
5 See D. Herlihy, *Medieval and Renaissance Pistoia: The Social History of an Italian Town, 1200–1430*, New Haven, Conn., 1967, pp. 240–50.

6 C. -M. de la Roncière, 'Pauvres et pauvreté à Florence au XIVe siècle', in M. Mollat (ed.) *Etudes sur l'histoire de la pauvreté*, 2 vols, Paris, 1974, vol. 2, pp. 684–95.

7 M. Villani, *Cronica*, Bk. 1, ch. 2; ed. F. G. Dragomanni, 2 vols, Florence, 1846, vol. 1, pp. 11–12.

8 See for example G. Brucker (ed. and trans.) *The Society of Renaissance Florence: A Documentary Study*, New York, 1971, pp. 229–31.

9 R. A. Goldthwaite, *The Building of Renaissance Florence: An Economic and Social History*, Baltimore, Md, 1980, pp. 335–40. Venice explicitly linked its public health concerns to the problem of depopulation; see for example M. Brunetti, 'Venezia durante la peste del 1348', *Ateneo veneto*, 1909, vol. 32.

10 A. G. Carmichael, *Plague and the Poor in Renaissance Florence*, Cambridge, 1986, esp. chs 4–5; J. Henderson, 'Epidemics in Renaissance Florence: medical theory and government response', in N. Bulst and R. Delort (eds) *Maladies et société (XIIe–XVIIIe siècles)*, Paris, 1988.

11 For example B. Grmek, 'Renfermement des pauvres en Italie (XIVe–XVIIe siècle): remarques préliminaires', in *Mélanges en l'honneur de Fernand Braudel*, 2 vols, Toulouse, 1973, vol. 1.

12 B. Cecchetti, 'La medicina in Venezia nel 1300', *Archivio veneto*, first series, 1883, vol. 26, pp. 85–8; G. Albini, *Guerra, fame, peste: crisi di mortalità e sistema sanitario nella Lombardia tardomedievale*, Bologna, 1982, ch. 2.

13 K. Park and J. Henderson, '"The first hospital among Christians": the Ospedali di Santa Maria Nuova in early sixteenth-century Florence', *Medical History*, 1991, vol. 35, p. 164.

14 Examples in Archivio di stato di Firenze: Provvisioni-Registri (hereafter PR)-38, fol. 57v; PR-41, fol. 38r. All archival references, unless otherwise stated, are to documents in the Archivio di stato di Firenze. On Urbino, Parma and other such cities, see V. Nutton, 'Continuity or rediscovery? The city physician in classical Antiquity and mediaeval Italy', in A. W. Russell (ed.) *The Town and State Physician in Europe from the Middle Ages to the Enlightenment*, Wolfenbüttel, 1981, p. 33.

15 See in general Nutton, op. cit., pp. 26–9; C. M. Cipolla, *Public Health and the Medical Profession in the Renaissance*, Cambridge, 1976, pp. 88–91. On Venice, R. Palmer, 'Physicians and the state in post-medieval Italy', in Russell (ed.) op. cit., p. 47.

16 PR-27, fol. 98r; also PR-23, fol. 12v, PR-32, fol. 105r (old num.); PR-27, fol. 98r; Statute of the Captain of the People of 1355, IV, 74 (Statuti del comune di Firenze-11, fol. 146v).

17 Details in K. Park, *Doctors and Medicine in Early Renaissance Florence*, Princeton, NJ, 1985, pp. 87–94.

18 See Park, 1985, op. cit., pp. 66–71.

19 R. Ciasca, *L'arte dei medici e speziali nella storia e nel commercio fiorentino dal secolo XII al XV*, Florence, 1927, pp. 295n, 299.

20 Park, 1985, op. cit., pp. 29–30, 107–10. Annual dues usually came to about two florins (roughly eight lire), which represented about sixteen days of work for a manual labourer in the construction industry; see Goldthwaite, op. cit., pp. 322–5.

21 L. Passerini, *Storia degli stabilimenti di beneficenza e d'istruzione elementare gratuita della città di Firenze*, Florence, 1853, p. 488; F. Carabellese, 'Le condizioni dei poveri a Firenze nel secolo XIV', *Rivista storica italiana*, 1895, vol. 12, p. 417.

22 See J. Henderson, 'The parish and the poor in Florence at the time of the Black Death: the case of S. Frediano', in J. Henderson (ed.) 'Charity and the poor in medieval and Renaissance Europe', *Continuity and Change*, 1988, vol. 3.

23 See in general J. Henderson, 'The hospitals of late medieval and Renaissance Florence: a preliminary survey', in L. Granshaw and R. Porter (eds) *Hospitals in History*, London, 1989; also Passerini, op. cit.; A. d'Addario, *Aspetti della contrariforma a Firenze*, Rome, 1972, ch. 2; M. A. Mannelli, 'Istituzione e soppressione degli ospedali minori in Firenze', *Studi di storia ospitaliera*, 1956, vol. 3.

24 P. R. Gavitt, *Charity and children in Renaissance Florence: the Ospedale degli Innocenti, 1410–1536*, Ann Arbor, Michigan, 1990, C. Trexler, 'The foundlings of Florence, 1395–1455', *History of Childhood Quarterly*, 1973, vol. 1; R. C. Trexler, 'A widows' asylum of the Renaissance: the Orbatello of Florence', in P. N. Stearns (ed.) *Old Age in Preindustrial Society*, New York, 1982. Details on the other hospitals in the works cited in the preceding note and in contemporary tax surveys: see for example Catasto-185, 190, 194, 195, 291, 292, 293 (1427–9), and Decima della repubblica-66, 67, 68, 69, 70 (1495).

25 Catasto-185, fol. 626r.

26 Passerini, op. cit., pp. 125–35; M. A. Mannelli, 'L'ospedale di S. Antonio in Firenze', *Ospedali d'Italia, Chirurgia*, 1965, vol. 12.

27 In addition to the general references above, see Park and Henderson, op. cit.; G. Pampaloni, *Lo spedale di Santa Maria Nuova*, Florence, 1961, ch. 1; R. Goldthwaite and W. R. Rearick, 'Michelozzo and the Ospedale di San Paolo in Florence', *Mitteilungen des Kunsthistorischen Institutes von Florenz*, 1977, vol. 21; B. J. Trexler, 'Hospital patients in Florence: San Paolo, 1567–68', *Bulletin of the History of Medicine*, 1974, vol. 48; E. Coturri, 'L'ospedale così detto "di Bonifazio" in Firenze', *Pagine di storia della medicina*, 1959, vol. 3; M. A. Mannelli, 'L'ospedale di San Matteo in Firenze', *Ospedali d'Italia, Chirurgia*, 1964, vol. 11.

28 Statements based on a selection of the hospital account books, including Santa Maria Nuova (hereafter SMN)-4408, 4437, 4453, 4458, 4477, 4479, 4495, and (for the contents of the pharmacy) L. Chiappelli and A. Corsini, 'Un antico inventario dello spedale di S. M. Nuova in Firenze (a. 1376)', *Rivista delle biblioteche e degli archivi*, 1921, vol. 32.

29 For example Biblioteca nazionale di Firenze: MS. Magl. XV, 92, fols 44v, 190r.

30 Statute of 1374: preserved in an Italian summary and transcribed in Passerini, op. cit., pp. 839–50 (original in SMN-10, fols 14v–26v). Statute sent to Henry VII: transcribed in Passerini, op. cit., pp. 851–67, and translated in Park and Henderson, op. cit.

31 Statute in Park and Henderson, op. cit., ch. 21.

32 SMN-3, *ad annum* 1421; SMN-10, fol. 12v.

33 SMN-31, fols 4r, 6r.
34 Statute in Park and Henderson, op. cit., chs 21 and 30.
35 When San Bastiano finally opened in 1494, it was administered largely by the devotional and charitable Company of the Misericordia: Henderson, 1989, op. cit., pp. 106–10.
36 On these doctors and on the organization of the medical profession in Florence, see Park, 1985, op. cit., ch. 1 and Index of Doctors and their Families.
37 Cipolla, op. cit., p. 4; E. Coturri, 'La scuola di Santa Maria Nuova di Firenze', *Ospedali d'Italia, Chirurgia*, 1964, vol. 10. E. Coturri, 'Le scuole ospedaliere di chirurgia del granducato di Toscana (secc. XVII–XIX)', *Minerva medica*, 1958, vol. 49.
38 The following discussion is based on the books of the dead of Santa Maria Nuova, SMN-730 (women 1474–94), 731 (men 1503–12), 732 (women 1495–1500, very incomplete), 733 (men 1513–28), 734 (women 1518–27), 735 (men 1527–8), 736 (women 1527–30), 737 (men 1528–32); and the books of the sick of San Paolo, Ospedali riuniti-San Paolo-640 (men 1554–61), 889 (men 1562–8); and B. J. Trexler, op. cit.
39 The rates for individual years ranged from a high of 12.3 per cent in 1512 to a low of 7.6 per cent in 1519.
40 The rates for individual years ranged from a high of 6.5 per cent in 1554 to a low of 4.1 per cent in 1559.
41 Figures for Santa Maria Nuova based on a sample of patients who died between August 1518 and July 1519 chosen because that is the only year that provides comparable information for women; those for San Paolo based on the year 1554, chosen because the records for that year contain discharge dates for men who did not die. The breakdown for these two years is as follows:

Santa Maria Nuova (1518–19)

Length of stay (in days)	Men		Women	
	Number	% of men in sample	Number	% of total women
1–10	134	58	101	36
11–20	27	12	61	22
21–40	41	18	38	14
41–100	22	10	48	17
101–200	6	2	22	8
201–800	—	—	9	3
Total	230	100	279	100

San Paolo (1554, men only)

	Dead		Discharged	
	Number	% of total dead	Number	% of total discharged
1–10	17	68	140	63
11–20	6	24	73	33
21–40	2	8	8	4
Total	25	100	221	100

42 B. J. Trexler, op. cit., p. 54. See Risse, op. cit., pp. 46–7, for other reasons for discharge.

43 Based on the figures in B. J. Trexler, op. cit., pp. 45–50, revised and corrected with reference to the discussion of diagnoses and causes of death in Carmichael, op. cit., pp. 35–54.

44 From August 1528 to July 1529, the only year for which admission numbers were recorded for women, the hospital took in 2,780 female patients, as opposed to 5,187 men; during that year, roughly 26 per cent of the women died, as opposed to about 17 per cent of the men. (This was a time of plague; both the mortality rates and the admission totals are atypically high and a poor basis for generalization.)

45 See figures in note 41.

46 Henry Piers noted that in 1595 the male beds held two patients and the female beds held three: E. P. de G. Chaney, '"Philanthropy in Italy": English observations on Italian hospitals, 1545–1789', in T. Riis (ed.) *Aspects of Poverty in Early Modern Europe*, Florence, 1981, p. 191.

47 Carmichael, op. cit., pp. 37–9.

48 See note 24. There is no evidence that the women's hospital acted as a maternity ward, unlike the hospital of the Innocenti, which was in constant need of wet-nurses; see Gavitt, op. cit., p. 164.

49 N. Falcucci, *Sermones medicales septem*, S. I, t. 1, ch. 4, 4 vols, Venice, vol. 1, fol. 2vb. See L. Demaitre, 'Nature and the art of medicine in the later Middle Ages', *Mediaevalia*, 1976, vol. 2.

50 See N. G. Siraisi, *Taddeo Alderotti and his Pupils: Two Generations of Italian Medical Learning*, Princeton, NJ, 1981, pp. 290–302.

51 Biblioteca nazionale di Firenze: MS. Magl. XV, 92, fols 31v, 55r.

52 For example Grmek, op. cit., and I. Naso, *Medici e strutture sanitarie nella società tardo-medievale; il Piemonte dei secoli XIV e XV*, Milan, 1982.

53 See Henderson, 1989, op. cit.; Coturri, 'I più antichi provvedimenti adottati in Firenze per l'isolamento degli appestati', *Castalia*, 1959, vol. 15.

54 See C. Carpaneto da Langasco, *Gli spedali degli incurabili*, Genoa, 1938.

55 SMN-Incurabili-1, pp. 29–31, 36.

56 B. J. Trexler, op. cit., pp. 47–9; see also SMN-Incurabili-1, ch. 6; d'Addario, op. cit., p. 95.

57 Naso, op. cit., pp. 28–9, 35.

58 See d'Addario, op. cit., pp. 74–92; D. Lombardi, 'Poveri a Firenze:

programmi e realizzazioni della politica assistenziale dei Medici tra cinque e seicento', in G. Politi *et al.* (eds) *Timore e carità; i poveri nell'Italia moderna*, Cremona, 1982; B. Pullan, *Rich and Poor in Renaissance Venice: the Social Institutions of a Catholic State, to 1620*, Oxford, 1971, esp. pp. 213–38.

3

THE MOTIVATIONS OF BENEFACTORS

An overview of approaches to the study of charity

Sandra Cavallo

The ideas in this chapter originate within the framework of my study of a charitable system, operating in Turin, capital of the Duchy, then the Kingdom of Savoy, between the late sixteenth and the end of the eighteenth centuries. My attempt to reconstruct the development of forms of assistance towards the poor and the sick, and the methods of regulating and financing charities over this broad time-span, has highlighted the weakness of arguments normally used to explain charitable behaviour and poor relief. The explanatory models most commonly employed to analyse new poor relief initiatives, new categories of the assisted and new representations of poverty were unable satisfactorily to explain the changes which I observed, such as fluctuations in the trend of charitable bequests and changes in attitudes towards different institutions and measures.

The case of Turin appears first of all to be out of line with a religious chronology which regards the principal turning-points in attitudes towards the poor and in charitable behaviour as being the Counter-Reformation and, conversely, the 'dechristianization' and secularization of control over assistance. It is noticeable that religiously based explanations tend to be seen as decisive above all in the study of Catholic countries. Although the tendency to regard European systems of poor relief as an expression of the Protestant (or Catholic) ethic and to postulate the superiority of the former has been rejected in recent years, it is clear that a move away from the interpretation of attitudes towards the poor in religious terms has been achieved only in the study of the English case. Indeed the same studies that criticize the Catholic/Protestant distinction still in fact accept a confessional image of Catholic societies and still attribute a central role to the activity of the church and to religious sentiments in determining poor-relief measures.[1] It is symptomatic that the work of Michel Vovelle, which of all works in recent years has most influenced studies of charity in a Catholic context, views charitable bequests precisely as a barometer of piety.[2] Yet it would quite evidently be unthinkable to apply such an interpretation to the case of England, where even though religious affiliation is regarded as having a considerable influence on charitable behaviour, it is evaluated in its social and political as well as its doctrinal dimensions.

The case of Turin cannot therefore be fitted within the paradigm established by Vovelle and accepted by the majority of subsequent studies. Private charity here displays a quite specific trend: it remained a marginal phenomenon for a long period, during which time the funding of the poor relief system derived essentially from the municipal budget (as well as from income from the ancient patrimony of the hospitals). Bequests and donations began to become an important resort for the hospitals and other institutions of assistance only in the last years of the seventeenth century. But above all the greatest development of private charity (both in terms of the number of bequests and donations and also of the total amount of money given out in charitable initiatives) took place in the middle decades of the eighteenth century, when we ought to be observing the effects of dechristianization. In this period, moreover, the absorption by the state of control over the institutions of assistance was taking place, so there is all the more reason why we should expect to find a decline of private charity in favour of forms of centralized intervention.

The trend of charity in Turin does not become any more coherent if we try to understand it as a reflection of different images of poverty which might emerge alongside not only the evolution of religious sentiment but also more complex changes in ideology. Changes in the form of poor relief have often been viewed as developing through different models of intervention that reflect the establishment of various ways of seeing and perceiving the poor. Thus one can identify periods in which the prevalent tendency was either to isolate and confine the poor, or to exploit them as a cheap labour force. Equally there were periods in which support shifted from institutional to home relief, or from more generalized forms of relief to medical charities and to the treatment of illness. In reality, the development of the behaviour of benefactors does not reflect a clear change in preferences. If we follow the transformations of a particular system of poor relief over time, it is clear that the various models of assistance coexist or at least recur spasmodically and with renewed intensity within a given period. Rather than seek a determinate transition from one pattern to another, as has generally been done, it seems necessary to come to terms with a much more complex picture of the different meanings taken on by recurring and apparently similar forms of relief. Moreover, the typological classification usually adopted is of little use. It is difficult to trace a coherent line of development in relation to a particular type of institution or provision for the poor (for example 'hospitals for the sick'). Each institution has in fact a strong individual identity, a life and a logic of development all its own, which can only partly be traced back to a pattern common to the category to which it nominally belongs.

It is difficult, for example, to identify a common pattern of development or chronology in the history of the three general hospitals for the sick located in Turin. The Osdepale di S. Maurizio e Lazzaro, created in 1575, was for a long period an almost entirely nominal presence within the city. It acquired a role as a centre of assistance to the sick only in the middle of the seventeenth century, when it increased in size, growing from fourteen beds in 1656 to fifty beds at the end of the century. At this point, however, it became virtually paralysed, and remained stagnant and neglected by private charity for the whole of the following century. The Ospedale di S. Giovanni di Dio, created in 1597 by the hospital order of the Brothers of Charity (who also managed the great and highly popular Milan hospital), maintained an extremely marginal role throughout its existence, and was never able to establish itself or to obtain support from benefactors. A century after its creation, the hospital still had only ten beds. In the following century, the Brothers abandoned their establishment definitively and left the city. The fortunes of the Ospedale Maggiore di S. Giovanni Battista were different again. Of ancient origin, the institution attracted bequests and donations from the 1540s which allowed it to emerge from a long period of crisis to establish itself as a major centre for urban poor relief. The great charitable impulse behind its development took place, however, only from the last decades of the seventeenth century. Indeed thanks to the generosity of its benefactors it was able to set about the construction of a large new building in 1680. It expanded uninterruptedly throughout the following century, growing from 36 beds in the middle of the seventeenth century to 242 beds in 1730, and it was able to accommodate about 500 sick people at the end of the eighteenth century. To understand this wide range of developments, we must consider therefore what the hospitals represented over and above their common identity as medical institutions. In reality, what mattered in the eyes of contemporaries was less the type of relief activity which occurred within such institutions than the social milieux from which their governors were drawn (such as the court circles, the magistracy or the City Council). It is the latter which is the decisive factor in explaining the different favours accorded them by benefactors.

An approach which seeks to provide an explanation of oscillations in charitable activity on the basis of economic trends also comes up against some major contradictions. In analogous circumstances of economic depression or prosperity very different reactions on the part of benefactors occur. Indeed in studies of charity, reference to the economic situation seems an ambivalent argument, since it is used to explain contrary trends in charitable development. The lack of cogency of such patterns is clearly visible in comparisons over lengthy periods. We see this, for example, in a work on testamentary charity in Nîmes and Lyon, where it is stated:

> In the 1630s, the continuing decline of purchasing power, in addition to high taxes, famines and riots aggravated the need of the poor. . . . The acute needs of the poor stimulated the greatest outpouring of testamentary charity of the century.

Yet some decades later

> The famine and calamities of 1693–5 slightly reduced testamentary charity. . . . During the next two decades the silk industry prospered enough to reduce the need for charity [but] the decline in the silk industry in the 1670s produced a further decline in charity. . . . [And again] the economic and religious turmoil of the 1680s, caused by wars and the revocation of the Edict of Nantes . . . reduced the silk industry still further but so intensified religious feeling that the result was a noticeable increase in the mention of charity in wills.[3]

It is evident that the linkage between charitable trends and economic fluctuations is rather uncertain; the logical contradiction which such arguments run up against is then resolved by adducing an explanatory element hitherto absent, namely religious sentiment.

Of course the economic situation, along with other factors which more directly influenced the conditions of the poor and their state of need, is an essential constitutive element of the context in which charitable behaviour took place, but it is certainly not always as decisive in itself as is often assumed. As Hilary Marland has clearly pointed out:

> There was no obvious reason why a dispensary should have been set up in Wakefield in this particular year. There was no significant increase in the population of the town in the late eighteenth century and no noticeable deterioration in the health of the inhabitants (marked, for example, by an increase in epidemic disease or in industrial accidents). However its establishment did coincide with a discernible fall in living standards and an era of depression. Medical services for the poor of Wakefield meanwhile were lacking just as much as elsewhere.[4]

Recognizing the impossibility of identifying among the classic contextual factors a single explanatory element, Marland opts for an 'open' explanation in which she insists upon the complexity of the variables which could affect the decision to establish a dispensary.

It is certainly not my intention to criticize such approaches nor to return to a rigidly monocausal model. I would, however, like to suggest that the explanatory limits indicated above partly derive from the very nature of the variables most commonly utilized in the analysis of charitable change, which tend to confine the explanation within a single paradigm. Although interpretations of the charitable act have become very complex, the tendency to see charity as dependent on the conditions of the poor, and on the structure and development of poverty undoubtedly remains prevalent. Thus the analysis normally accords a central role to demographic or economic factors (prices, epidemics, famines, population growth, demographic crises, immigration, structure of occupations, etc.) which precisely enlarge or restrict the dimensions of poverty and modify its characteristics. Charity, that is, is interpreted essentially as a *response* to the needs of the poor or to the threat they represent. It should indeed be pointed out that even in studies which highlight the aim of benefactors to exhibit paternalism, to seek consensus, or to establish social control, a similar paradigm is present: concern for the situation of the poor – whether this gives rise to pity or on the contrary to fear – is seen as the motivating element behind charitable action. In other words, existing studies tend to give priority to arguments based on *demand*, and this inhibits exploration of other kinds of explanations, relatively independent of the needs of the poor, but linked rather to the multiple meanings which charity held for benefactors.

The fact that the individuals involved in the management and funding of charity were motivated principally by concern for the poor is not in any way discounted. What remains to be demonstrated is whether what we see as the clear and evident consequences of charitable activity was the intention – and the main intention – that motivated benefactors. As often happens, historians arbitrarily establish a link of direct intentionality between the object of their research – in this case a certain charitable form or institution – and the action which generated it – in this case the charitable act. Such a procedure takes for granted a direct link between intention and consequences. It avoids a less literal analysis of the reasons behind charitable behaviour which takes into account its symbolic and metaphorical meanings. It seems clear to me, however, that people often engaged in charity as a result of concerns other than those generated by thoughts of the poor, and that the reconstruction of these concerns could provide an important explanatory element in the analysis of charitable trends, their acceleration or immobilism, their frequent inconsistencies compared to the development of poverty. One must therefore concentrate on the motivations of individuals and consider the impulse which moves people to give, through a particular form of poor relief and at a particular moment.

The subjective experience of individuals involved in charity is generally unknown. Individuals are usually viewed as instruments for the realization of schemes aimed at consoling the poor in their misery, at educating and moralizing them, or at rendering them dependent and controllable. The tendency to neglect the level of individual motivation for charity is not just characteristic of works which concentrate on the investigation of the conditions of poverty and relations between rich and poor.[5] This lack of interest occurs too in works – relatively separate from the first group – which view changing ideas concerning the poor as the principal motor of assistance.[6] In the first kind of study, there is, as I have suggested, the danger of a functionalist interpretation, in which charitable action is understood essentially as a response to the conditions of the poor and as a force counterbalancing social tension. In studies which concentrate on changes in ideologies concerning the poor, on the other hand, charitable activity is viewed as a mechanical transposition of prevalent doctrines of political economy or of the ethics associated with different religious beliefs. In this approach, there is clearly too strong a view of ideology or religious culture as determinate, and in addition an idealization of social behaviour as something which is governed only by considerations of economic rationality or public utility, and not at all by the interests, emotions and conflicts within which social actors operate. That is to say, these studies do not concern themselves with the relationship between emergent and different definitions and images of poverty and the realm of immediate meanings with which charitable action towards the poor was invested for the individuals directly involved in charitable activity. There is no attempt to explore, in other words, the way in which subjectivity contributed to the formation of ideologies about the poor.

That involvement in charity was sought partly out of concern for individuals' own position in power or status has often been noted. It is almost commonplace to observe that the charitable impulse was motivated by aims which were secular and which involved personal rewards. Generally, however, this point is hinted at only sporadically, as if to show the historian's common sense and lack of naïvety. The quest for prestige and influence is considered as an essential element in charitable action, but an element without a history, being integral to human nature. It is not contextualized and there is no attempt to ask how far it is specific to the situation under review. It is, moreover, noticeable that the secular values of charitable action are easily recognized in the context of biographical analysis,[7] but that this analytical dimension gets lost, in favour of more dignified explanations, when the object under review becomes charity as a social phenomenon.

Recent studies, particularly those relating to England, have however shown greater concern with these mechanisms and they suggest how involvement in a charitable initiative could play an important part in relationships between elites. It has been shown how participation in the management of hospitals and other structures of poor relief favoured the creation of networks of interest allowing the establishment of contacts, business links and influence over work and career opportunities. The post of benefactor or governor also offered obscure individuals, perhaps excluded from other jobs within the public sphere, the possibility of obtaining and exercising patronage.[8] Above all, these studies have started to root charitable action in a specific political scenario: to see it, for example, in relation to the opposition between urban elites and landowners, or to the rivalry between different factions of the urban elite or, on the other hand, to the need to create common objectives and integrative mechanisms after a long period of division and conflict.[9] They have thus begun to establish a link between the timing of power conflicts and charitable initiatives. This analytical approach has been developed in the work of Stephen Macfarlane on the London Corporation of the Poor, and above all in that of Timothy Hitchcock on the workhouse movement, where this approach frames the entire investigation. These studies show how action to reform the existing system of poor relief and the initiatives which led to the foundation of workhouses and charity schools in many English communities and parishes in the late seventeenth and eighteenth centuries, were heavily motivated by the intention of shifting management of assistance to social and political groups other than those which administered the poor rates or held control of local government. The charitable initiative is thus analysed as a vehicle of political disputes and as a means of modifying the power balance.[10] As Stephen Macfarlane summarizes: 'late Stuart debates on the poor were thus as much about *who* ought to govern indigent or able-bodied paupers as *how* they should be governed'.[11]

Such an approach, which reverses the perspective from which the charitable phenomenon is normally analysed, has important methodological and interpretative implications. Charity, normally considered as an expression of policies towards the poor, is broadly portrayed as politics between elites. It becomes a question of widening the perspective, hitherto restricted essentially to the analysis of changes in the attitudes of the rich towards the poor, to include conflicts which pervaded the upper orders and changes in the definition of the stratification of elites which found expression in charitable activity. In this light, the studies just cited have limits. While interpreting charity as an instrument of political strategy, they restrict themselves to the configurations of party and religious factions that such strategies could assume. It is clear that competition between individuals and among elite groups is not restricted to conflict between Whigs and Tories or between various sorts of Dissenters and Anglicans which often give rise to initiatives towards the poor.[12] The analysis of tensions, interests and ambitions that motivated benefactors and administrators to invest in charity is thus not developed to its full explanatory potential, and so does not provide an overall framework for the interpretation of charitable activity.

That behaviour towards the poor should be motivated by a secular logic does not mean that charity should be viewed as the result of clear-sighted calculation of maximizing one's own benefit. It often arose under the influence of a rhetoric and passwords whose ambiguous meaning is not easily decoded, and to which donors adhered on the wave of emotional stimuli. Ideologies exercised a considerable influence on charitable behaviour, even if this was revealed to be contrary to the interests of the social actors. It is, however, undeniable that such rhetoric and hierarchies of values did not arise out of nothing, but were derived from the reality of social conflicts, and that they constituted an articulation of the political discourse within which were negotiated the relationships between different segments of the elite as well as between rich and poor. The problem remains therefore of reconstructing the link between the emergence of specific ideas and measures towards the poor, and particular patterns of relationship and conflict. This has to be explored without negating the autonomy which such forms of ideology enjoyed, and without maintaining that their influence would have been restricted solely to legitimizing the relations which had generated them.

In my work on Turin, I take into consideration the development of two sets of relationships which could have important repercussions for charitable attitudes: on one hand the tensions affecting the urban elites, and thus the pressures on their stratification and on models for exercising power in the city; on the other hand, the conflict generated in the sphere of the aristocratic family by the redefinition of family roles and procedures governing inheritance and control over family patrimony.

There is in fact a strong correlation between the trend of charitable action and the chronology of political and family conflict. From the 1560s, for more than fifty years, for example, assistance to the poor seems to have been dominated by the clash between municipal authority and the power of the Duke, following the latter's restoration after thirty years of French occupation. In this phase, charitable initiatives seem not to have derived from individuals and groups but rather to have been monopolized by the two opposing groups, the City Council and the Duchy. In the first decades, the development of an extensive system of municipal poor relief, which provided aid to the poor and free medical assistance to the sick principally on a home-relief basis, seems to have been linked to the creation of a strong municipal identity, capable of successfully negotiating with the ducal power the recognition of a full set of privileges, fiscal exemptions and autonomy from the central government. In the thirty-year period from 1590 to 1620, charitable initiatives came in turn to signify open competition between the two authorities: rival institutions were established by a ducal authority in the process of consolidating itself, while each of the two powers sought to frustrate the initiatives of the other. The disputes about who should direct poor relief, and how, became continuous and violent.

For a long time therefore assistance to the poor was essentially a means of strengthening the identity, support and influence of the two centres of power contesting control of the city. But charitable activity did not always reflect a formal political entity. In other periods it was predominantly an expression of the action of individuals and families. The development of private charity occurred in Turin from the 1670s, a period in which the ritual and ceremonial space within the city came to be monopolized by the family of the sovereign and his expanding court. Donations and legacies grew in number at the same time as the emergence of forms of celebration praising donors' generosity. These included the practice of setting up a bust or a statue in the receiving institution and the diffusion of a series of rituals of gratitude which utilized the poor in choreographical fashion and which also constituted occasions for honouring the author of the charitable gesture and his lineage. These ritualistic and iconographical forms, hitherto limited to the more exclusive entourage of the Duke, were effectively democratized within charitable institutions offering an alternative ceremonial space to a broad range of elites excluded from civic rituals. Hospitals, rebuilt over these years in sumptuously baroque style, became the backdrop of civic prestige, and offered a symbolic confirmation of the intense processes of social ascent and formation of new wealth that were taking place in these years.

If in the years around the end of the seventeenth century, charity was motivated essentially by a quest for the symbolic confirmation of the status of the benefactor, in other periods it aimed at more tangible results. In the 1730s the charitable act became a vehicle for the privatization of poor relief: donations were no longer given unconditionally. In an increasing number of cases, they were subject to conditions imposed by benefactors, who determined who should benefit, and often entrusted control of the donations to the benefactors' own descendants or to particular bodies or organizations. Hospitals and other institutions became a resource for private influence, taking the form of *piazze* (the right to assign places in them) or of charitable funds controlled privately and targeted at specific areas of protection (the poor of a parish, of a certain guild, or even of a kinship network). This constituted a response of the non-bureaucratic elites to changes in the running of the institutions which, against strong resistance, passed into the hands of state functionaries in these years. The outcome of these attempts at centralization was thus the fragmentation of charity into micro-systems of tutelage which restricted access to relief to individuals within given networks of protection.

The fact that change occurred in the proponents of charitable activity – now formal power institutions, now families and individuals, now groups of solidarity – and in the motivations behind their investment in charity, had important consequences for the poor, in that these developments modified the opportunities offered by the charitable system. The models of direction of charitable resources that emerged in these diverse political patterns (more or less pluralistic, monopolistic, corporative) either enlarged or restricted the channels of access to poor relief, and modified the qualifications that the poor had to possess and the language of desert that they had to recite in order to be accepted.

Even the definition of the categories to be assisted and the boundaries of deserving poverty were closely related to the phases of the conflict between and within the elites. Periods of maximum tension within the elites led to the emergence of sets of values and rhetoric that often had a powerful impact upon the way in which the poor were viewed, and helped to establish new definitions of poverty. This was particularly evident in Turin during the long period of dispute between the Duchy and the municipality (1560s–1620s). In this period, the construction of the identity of the City Council rested on a rhetoric which associated dignity with the status of 'citizen', which aimed to legitimize the claims for autonomy on the part of the city and the particular privileges being won 'for the citizens'. In this context, attitudes towards the poor changed too, and rigid lines of demarcation were erected between citizens and outsiders. People from other parts of the Duchy, who (precisely because they had not long been resident in the city and were therefore without accommodation or relationships) had until a few years earlier been advantaged by provisions for relief, were now viewed as individuals who were depriving citizens of the resources for poor relief available in the city. In the initiatives towards the poor, the 'outsiders' were now the target of violent verbal attacks and with growing frequency they began to have extended to them measures of banishment from the city hitherto utilized only occasionally against 'outsiders' from other states.[13]

The 'citizen' became the privileged recipient of the relief provided by the City Council, although the definition of 'citizen' remained vague. When efforts were made to give concrete form to what had originally been only a propagandistic slogan, uncertain definitions resulted which were anyway extremely bland compared with the vehemence with which the privileges and exclusive rights were claimed on behalf of citizens. The citizen, it gradually emerged, was someone who had resided in the city either 'since last Christmas' or else 'since Michaelmas' – a definition which clearly included a majority of the temporary immigrants who had moved into the capital in the cold weather and during the cessation of agricultural work.

Soon the question of establishing a precise definition was deferred. Clearly the rhetoric of citizenship was essentially a weapon in political conflict. A strict definition would have meant, among other things, openly opposing the dynamic of the growth of the city, which was expanding in these years, and acquiring the status of capital thanks precisely to the establishment in the city of immigrants who in other respects had been encouraged to move in.[14] However, by the 1590s the distinction between city-dweller and outsider was established as the new language of discrimination applied to the poor and would remain one of the principal attributes of deserving poverty (with, however, varying intensity in comparison with other selection criteria) for the next two centuries. Equally the practice of banishing the undeserving poor from the city became a typical measure to which recourse was still made in the eighteenth century at times of major economic crisis and overcrowding.

The needs of political consolidation and conflict were thus the main motive force which led in the second half of the sixteenth century to the establishment of a complex system of assistance controlled by the City Council,[15] and to the creation of new attitudes and discriminatory principles towards the poor. The new models of relief thus emerged not so much as a response to pressure from below and to changing conditions of poverty but rather as the articulation of the City Council's political autonomy and the city-dweller's privileged identity. Thus the development of poor relief ideologies and practices cannot always be explained in functional terms or as the legitimation of a given model of relations between rich and poor. Often, the form assumed by ideas on the poor can be explained as the metaphorical transposition of relationships between the elites. The opposition between city-dweller and outsider that shaped policies towards the poor between the end of the sixteenth and the beginning of the seventeenth centuries was precisely a symbolic expression of conflict between two differing political spheres and different models for the exercise of power. It was not by chance that the ducal offensive against municipal prerogatives – of which poor relief was a preferred terrain – should be conducted a few decades later on the same metaphorical level: a rhetoric of universal and indiscriminate charity directed to all 'subjects' was contrasted with the City Council's practice of limiting relief to city-dwellers, a policy now vigorously attacked as pitiless and contrary to the exigencies of Christian charity.

Initiatives towards the poor may also thus be viewed as a secondary result of, or a vehicle for, tensions within the elites. We see this again in the middle decades of the seventeenth century, when charitable activity appeared to be dominated by female beneficence, and was directed particularly towards the more difficult circumstances of the female condition. Women, especially widows, the *malmaritate* (that is victims of turbulent marital relationships), women abandoned by or separated from their husbands, along with unmarried women, temporarily became the object of particular interest and appropriate institutions and measures were established in their favour. In this case too, the identification of new categories of the deserving poor does not reflect a worsening of the phenomenon of female solitude but seems rather to constitute the means of expressing a rhetoric of female weakness. This was closely connected to conflicts relating to the strengthening of primogeniture and to practices which aristocratic families were developing at this time connected with the control and transmission of property which were unfavourable to women. The measures regarding the poor thus appear part of the construction of a discourse of female vulnerability that was emerging out of the difficult change from lineage to family, a discourse which concerned charitable donors, rather than the objects of their charity.

One may object that these forms of assistance were not new. In many charitable systems, for example, the citizen and the widow were considered privileged targets of charitable activity. The fact that these models were imitated from outside or even derived from the city's own past, after a period of stagnation, does not, however, diminish the relevance of understanding why they re-emerged and grew so strong in this particular period. It was anyway the context of local changes at work which attributed new force and contemporary meaning to these established languages of discrimination.

The centrality which I am here according to conflict inside the elite as the moving force behind poor relief may appear to be a return to 'history from above'. From such a viewpoint it might appear that the poor lose any role in the definition of poor relief policies, even the classic one of arousing fear and defensiveness. I would not, however, wish to deny the powerful pressure which the poor can exert on charitable activity. In particular, the model of reciprocity proposed by E. P. Thompson as a key to the understanding of the relationship between the elite and the labouring classes allows us to explore the charitable act as the consequence of an exchange relationship, and one of negotiation between rich and poor.[16]

However, the dynamics of vertical relationships between rich and poor are not the only forces in play in charitable activity, nor do they entirely explain its chronology. It is true that in some periods poor relief may be predominantly shaped by the need to provide a direct response to pressing problems of public order and impoverishment. In the latter half of the eighteenth century, for example, the redrawing of the poor relief system in Turin seems to have been largely determined by the alarming level of social conflict and by the emergence of a different structure of urban poverty. The scale of the economic crisis, of rural exodus and unemployment, brought to the forefront social categories hitherto excluded from relief (adult males and able-bodied young men) who became the target of particular apprehension and specific measures. Closely examined, however, not even in these years were changes in the character of poverty completely separate from changes that were modifying power relationships among the elites. Indeed, a weakening of vertical links of protection and of interdependence between the labouring classes and the upper classes is the consequence of the process of centralization of power in the hands of professionalized state functionaries – a process which drastically reduced the possibility, for large segments of the elite, of exercising patronage. This closure of the channels of reciprocity was largely responsible for the turbulence of these years, and for the particularly devastating impact of economic crisis and the changes in labour relations taking place in the countryside and in craft workshops.[17] The redefinition of relations between 'high' and 'low' observable in this period is thus only one aspect of a more complex process that also involved a transformation of patterns of power within the ruling classes.

By analysing changes in the patterns of power, we can thus provide a missing piece of the jigsaw. It allows us to recognize an essential factor of social dynamics and to explore how this interacts with other elements in play. This angle of vision also allows us to open up a direction for research which has been little utilized, namely the non-literal, symbolic meanings of the charitable act. The relationships and conflicts between the elites are not the sole, nor even the prime, explanatory element behind the development of forms of poor relief, but they do play a key role at certain moments. These dynamics seem to exert a considerable influence above all on the way models of relief and definitions of poverty are generated. This has been my emphasis in this chapter. If we turn from formulation to practice, the action of the poor becomes far more dominant, for they themselves utilized, reformulated and manipulated these models and languages.

NOTES

1 B. Pullan, *Rich and Poor in Renaissance Venice: The Social Institutions of a Catholic State, to 1620*, Oxford, 1971.

2 M. Vovelle, *Piété baroque et déchristianisation en Provence au XVIIIe siècle*, Paris, 1973.

3 W. J. Pugh, 'Catholics, Protestants and testamentary charity in seventeenth-century Lyon and Nîmes', *French Historical Studies*, vol. 11, 1980.

4 H. Marland, *Medicine and Society in Wakefield and Huddersfield, 1780–1870*, Cambridge, 1987, p. 123.

5 For a recent overview of studies on Britain, stressing social and economic approaches, see P. Slack, *Poverty and Policy in Tudor and Stuart England*, London, 1988. For other European countries see S. J. Woolf, *The Poor in Western Europe in the Eighteenth and Nineteenth Centuries*, London, 1986, introduction; and C. Jones, *The Charitable Imperative: Hospitals and Nursing in Ancien Régime and Revolutionary France*, London, 1989. One notes, however, that socio-economic elements have a less important part in studies on mainland Europe where explanations in which religious doctrines and state ideologies are seen

as the main motive force behind poor relief policies are dominant. See for example the works cited on Italy in M. Rosa, 'Chiesa, idee sui poveri e assistenza in Italia dal Cinque al Settecento', *Società e Storia*, 1980, vol. 10; B. Pullan, 'Support and redeem: charity and poor relief in Italian cities from the fourteenth to the seventeenth century', *Continuity and Change*, 1988, vol. 3; and my own remarks in S. Cavallo, 'Charity, power and patronage in eighteenth-century Italian hospitals: the case of Turin', in L. Granshaw and R. Porter (eds) *The Hospital in History*, London, 1989.

6 D. Owen, *English Philanthropy*, Cambridge, Mass., 1964; J. R. Poynter, *Society and Pauperism: English Ideas on Poor Relief, 1795–1834*, London, 1969; G. Himmelfarb, *The Idea of Poverty: England in the Early Industrial Age*, London, 1984.

7 For examples of how charitable activity is viewed within individual and family strategies see D. Cannadine, *Lords and Landlords: The Aristocracy and the Towns, 1774–1967*, Leicester, 1980; Cannadine (ed.) *Patricians, Power and Politics in Nineteenth-Century Towns*, Leicester, 1982. The treatment of the dynamics of charitable activity is more disappointing when the biography is that of a notable benefactor: see for example R. K. McClure, *Coram's Children: The London Foundling Hospital in the Eighteenth Century*, New Haven, Conn., 1981; and J. S. Taylor, *Jonas Hanway, Founder of the Marine Society: Charity and Policy in Eighteenth-Century Britain*, London, 1985.

8 For example L. Granshaw, *Saint Mark's Hospital, London: A Social History of a Specialist Hospital*, London, 1985, pp. 16–22; J. V. Pickstone, *Medicine and Industrial Society: A History of Hospital Development in Manchester and Its Region, 1752–1946*, Manchester, 1985, p. 11; G. B. Risse, *Hospital Life in Enlightenment Scotland: Care and Teaching at the Royal Infirmary of Edinburgh*, Cambridge, 1986, pp. 19, 28; Marland, op. cit., pp. 140–4; R. Porter, 'The gift relation: philanthropy and provincial hospitals in eighteenth-century England', in Granshaw and Porter, op. cit.; N. McKendrick, J. Brewer and J. H. Plumb, *The Birth of a Consumer Society: The Commercialisation of Eighteenth-Century Britain*, London, 1982, pp. 227–8.

9 D. Fraser, 'Voluntaryism and West Riding politics in the mid-nineteenth century', *Northern History*, 1976–7, vols 12–13; Porter, op. cit., and works cited by him on factional charity, pp. 151–5.

10 S. Macfarlane, 'Social policy and the poor in the late seventeenth century', in A. L. Beier and R. Finlay (eds) *The Making of the Metropolis: London, 1500–1700*, London, 1986; T. Hitchcock, 'The English workhouse: a study in institutional poor relief in selected counties, 1696–1750', D.Phil thesis, Oxford University, 1985. See also M. Fissell, 'The physic of charity: health and welfare in the West Country, 1690–1834', Ph.D thesis, University of Pennsylvania, 1988; and C. Rose, 'Politics at the London Royal Hospital, 1683–92' in Granshaw and Porter, op. cit.

11 Macfarlane, op. cit., p. 253.

12 The tendency to restrict analysis of political behaviour to its party political manifestations is an enduring characteristic of the English

historiographical tradition. See N. Landau, 'Eighteenth-century England: tales historians tell', *Eighteenth-Century Studies*, 1988–9, vol. 22, pp. 212–13, who proposes, in contrast, a return to a Namierite approach.

13 On these measures, see S. Cavallo, 'Patterns of poor relief and patterns of poverty in eighteenth-century Italy: the evidence of the Turin Ospedale di Carità', *Continuity and Change*, 1990, vol. 5.

14 The increase in Turin's population between 1571 and 1614 was 71 per cent, due mainly to immigration. On the formation of the capital, see G. Levi, 'Come Torino soffocò il Piemonte', in Levi, *Centro e periferia di uno stato assoluto: Tre saggi su Piemonte e Liguria in età moderna*, Turin, 1986, pp. 11–69.

15 At the end of the sixteenth century municipal councillors (together with the canons of the cathedral chapter, over whom they had a majority) managed the main hospital for the sick; they aided the poor through a system of home relief, and provided permits to beg for the non-able-bodied; they salaried a certain number of physicians and surgeons, who provided medical outdoor relief to the sick poor, plus a pharmacist who provided gratis the medicines required; they paid for the wet-nursing of foundlings; they gave charity secretly to the 'proud poor'; they hired a *Cavaliere di Virtù* (a sort of sheriff), who had the task of expelling the outside beggars in times of dearth.

16 E. P. Thompson, 'Eighteenth-century English society: class struggle without class?', *Social History*, 1978, vol. 3.

17 S. Cavallo, 'Conceptions of poverty and poor relief in Turin in the second half of the eighteenth century', in S. J. Woolf (ed.) *Domestic Strategies: Work and Family in France and Italy (17th–18th Centuries)*, Cambridge, 1991.

4

'HARDLY A HOSPITAL, BUT A CHARITY FOR PAUPER LUNATICS'?[1]

Therapeutics at Bethlem in the seventeenth and eighteenth centuries

Jonathan Andrews

The subject of charity inevitably provokes exhortation. Appropriately, then, I should like to begin this chapter by urging that the history of psychiatry has been coloured by a vituperative view which needs to be confronted more fully, if not abandoned altogether. This view, I would suggest, is largely the product of an overly retrospective and Whiggish historiography, which has failed to appreciate the pragmatics of psychiatric care in their proper context. The usual depiction of Bethlem Hospital, as an almshouse, or detention centre, rather than a centre of cure, belongs to this tradition, and although recently challenged, has remained particularly pervasive.[2] While this account may be accurate in many respects, its tone is misplaced and misleading, tending to denigrate the authenticity of the relief such institutions offered, and forging a somewhat anachronistic distinction between material and medical relief. Early modern charity embraced both these provisions. Even the modern concept of the hospital is not exclusionist, but is defined both as an 'institution providing medical and surgical treatment for persons ill or injured', and as a 'charitable institution' (*OED*). In fact, the way in which Bethlem functioned, even in its limited capacity as a charity dispensing material relief, has been little understood. Moreover, however ineffective we may judge the array of medicaments at Bethlem, it is simply erroneous to assert that the hospital was not concerned with therapeutics, and the cure of its patients; or, in other words, was not a hospital at all. In this chapter I have space to present only a selective outline of these issues, but one which I hope will posit some alternative ways of interpreting the type of care Bethlem dispensed.

In an age before state-funding, when hospitals relied for their survival on public benefactions, not just Bethlem, but all hospitals, had to be charities first and foremost. They were organized as charities and promoted themselves as charities. Governors gave their services gratis; subscribers often – in the eighteenth century, almost invariably – became governors; patients were admitted at reduced fees or gratis; many medical officers attended in a visiting, part honorary, capacity, only gradually becoming properly salaried and full-time employees. The 'Charge' that was read to each newly elected governor of Bridewell and Bethlem made manifest the philanthropic, quasi-religious sense in which each was to think of his office: namely as 'the distribucion [sic] of the Revenues designed by Charitable persons for . . . Excellent Ends', with a view to Judgement Day, when 'account will be taken of all the offices of Charity.'[3] From the 1640s onwards, Bethlem and the other great London hospitals[4] advertised themselves in unison at the annual Spital services as charities worthy of public contributions.[5] It was no empty claim on the governors' part that the ordinary revenues of Bethlem did not amount 'to two thirds p[ar]t of their yearly charge'.[6] Benefactors were vital to the extensiveness of a hospital's relief. For most of the eighteenth century, curable patients were maintained at Bethlem without any weekly charges, and incurables at only 2s. 6d., and these low rates were directly linked by the governors to the generosity of their benefactors.[7] Bethlem was largely dependent on the generosity of benefactors to finance its two great projects of expansion, in this period: the rebuilding at Moorfields, in 1675–6, and the new Incurables Establishment, of 1723–35; and yet was still forced to borrow substantially for the completion of both projects.[8] Just how difficult it was to keep hospitals solvent, at this time, needs to be appreciated. The overwhelming preoccupation of the administrative records of Bethlem with money matters – with assessing and obtaining debts from tenants, executors and sureties – is comprehensible only in this light. While such concerns obviously diverted the governors' attention from the actual health of their charges, Bethlem was hardly unique in this, as a cursory glance at the records of other hospitals is enough to establish. Moreover, it was to a considerable extent through the hospital's very success as a charity that Bethlem was able to achieve the financial security necessary to improve facilities, and to concentrate on therapeutic reforms.

The necessity of attracting donors' charity obviously influenced and compromised the type of care any charitable foundation dispensed, or claimed it was dispensing, during this period. Moreover, if hospitals were thoroughly negotiated entities, some were certainly more negotiated than others. Significantly many of the new eighteenth-century foundations sought an enhanced financial (and thus administrative) independence, through the longer-term investment of subscribers, citing the experience of older institutions like Bridewell and Bethlem (with their prodigious, but largely honorary, non-contributing boards of governors) which had remained too dependent on occasional benefactions and continuous fund-raising.[9] In particular, as it was uniquely exposed to the public eye as a resort for visitors, Bethlem's charity was influenced by a greater range of pressures than any other contemporary hospital. Thus it was that the public, not the patients, were so often at the forefront of its governors' minds; as, typically, in 1641, when expressing their anxiety over the sickness of two basketmen in the hospital, 'that much Charity was lost for want of good lookeing after it and attendinge it'.[10] The public relations aspect of charity, whereby hospitals projected themselves into the market-place, is nowhere more apparent in this period than in the rebuilding of Bethlem at Moorfields, when the governors paid more respect to 'the Grace & Ornament of the said Intended Building' (i.e. as rhetoric on behalf of the public, and of their own status) than to its therapeutic purpose, or even to the comfort of the patients.[11] Yet here it is context that is crucial. We should not expect seventeenth- or eighteenth-century hospitals to be purpose-built in the modern sense, nor, indeed, that the patients at Bethlem should be any more the dominant interest of governing elites, than were the patients of other contemporary hospitals.

Moreover, the concerns of the dispensers of charity and the needs of the objects of charity (medical or otherwise), were neither in perpetual opposition nor uniform in themselves. For example, while many supporters of Bridewell and Bethlem sought social and political status through civic duty, or through the display of their beneficence (most explicitly, on the tables listing benefactors hung up at the hospitals), others made anonymous donations or made emphatic statements of personal sympathies. The legacy of the long-serving governor Thomas Nixon at the end of the eighteenth century, which was confined exclusively to curable patients and bemoaned the 'perverting [of] that Hospital into an Alms House of incurable patients' says as much about the changing nature of charity at Bethlem (which had long catered for the chronically insane), as it does about its traditional combination of aims: how the hospital was able to incorporate a commitment to both the care and cure of illness, as well as the often divergent aims of its adherents. Even in characterizing Bethlem as an almshouse, Nixon recognized that the hospital had always been, and still was, concerned with the 'Cure' of its patients. Indeed he claimed to have been 'a joyfull Spectator of many Lunaticks who have been restored to their Senses by God's Blessing on the means and Assistance afforded them'.[12] Nixon was far from the only governor or benefactor of Bethlem who rejected a material or custodial notion of Bethlem's function, by excluding incurables from his donation.

There is, nevertheless, much evidence throughout the period to support the notion of Bethlem as best viewed as a dispenser of charity rather than simply of medicine. The hospital was anxious in fact to present itself in this fashion. Patients were admitted only if poor, upon petitions detailing their indigent circumstances, and provided that they were explicitly adjudged 'fitt obiect[s] of [the] Charity' of the hospital.[13] They were normally rejected or discharged if found of sufficient capacity to be supported elsewhere. Indeed until the earlier seventeenth century, the inmates of the hospital are collectively referred to (alongside those of Bridewell) in the Court of Governors' Minutes, as simply 'the poore' and occasionally as 'the prisoners'. Thereafter they are generally called 'the Lunatickes'. The term 'patient' was not regularly employed at Bethlem until the eighteenth century.[14] It was also not until the early seventeenth century that a medical staff was appointed to the hospital. The governors speak more emphatically in admission orders and elsewhere of the 'relief' of their charges than of their 'cure'. The contemporary notion of charity was all-embracing; 'Phisicke, dyett & lodging', and 'cure' itself, were regarded as but components of this charitable relief which Bethlem conferred on its patients. Occasionally bedding, clothing, burial, transportation and, invariably, the fee levied for the maintenance of patients were treated as part of Bethlem's relief. The weekly fee was described as a payment 'towards the charge of his/her keeping', signifying that it was not sufficient to defray all expenses incurred, but was a charitable concession, and that the charity of Bethlem was to supply the residue. Some patients, usually vagrants bereft of friends or means, were supported completely on the charity of the hospital, down to the clothes on their backs. The obligors[15] of most patients were able to make individual bargains with the Court of Governors, by outlining their conditions of poverty, and could subsequently obtain abatements of their original fees by further petitions proving their decayed state. Thus it was primarily on the material circumstances of the insane and their obligors that eligibility, the settling of charges and the actual bond of performance were based. Primitive prognostic and diagnostic criteria existed, such as the duration of a patient's affliction, but these took second place (as perhaps did the interests of the afflicted themselves) to the interests of their friends or parish, who sought to ease the burden on themselves. While Bethlem was the preferred choice of many (metropolitan) families and most parishes, this was less because of its promise of a remedy than because it was simply cheaper than a private mad-house or even, at times, than boarding-out in the community.

However, we must be careful not to underestimate the sympathetic spirit of the relief that Bethlem (and like institutions) dispensed. Many families and parishes were simply unable (or even unwilling) to cater for their distressed members and would have been unable to support them in Bethlem, without the charitable mitigations of the administration there. In the 1650s Martha Boutha, for example, was granted an abatement of the fee for her niece, who had 'beene long Lunatique' in Bethlem, being herself 'a poore Widd[ow]' and 'able to pay the same noe longer'.[16] The compassionate tenor of other entries in the Court Minutes, like that concerning the petition of Benjamin Hide, for the continuance of his son in Bethlem, is overt: Hide's weekly fee is reduced to just 2s. 6d., in respect of his 'being decayed in his estate' and 'this Courte comisserating his sad condic[i]on'.[17] What followers of Foucault might prefer to interpret as coercive, street-cleaning tendencies behind the confinement in Bethlem during 1655 of vagrants like Sarah King, described as 'crazed and distracted . . . taken up in the streetes of this Citty', might just as easily be interpreted as affordable provision made in the face of neglect.[18] It is in this light also that the typical petition for the reception of Mary Calling, in Bethlem, may be viewed, she being described by her fellow parishioner in 1651 as 'a poore distracted woman lying in the streetes there'.[19]

Assuredly, like most contemporary hospitals, Bethlem functioned, to some degree, as an extension of the embracing, and sometimes coercive, arm of poor relief. The vast majority of patients received by the hospital were supported by parishes on the poor rate and conveyed to, and represented at, the Court by parish officers, or were supported by poor individuals and families who were not quite poor enough to be relieved by their parishes. There is an element of bullying in the way families and parishes were required to give security to collect and provide for patients once discharged and were sued if they failed to do so, and in the way they were summoned to the Court, either to become bound for the maintenance of the insane at Bethlem or to provide for them instead themselves.[20] Yet the hospital also operated in a more positive way, reminding them of their duties to care for the insane. In cases like that of John Sanderson, a poor Leicester lunatic with 'noe freinds or means', the Court can be seen to be acting explicitly in both these capacities. By addressing a letter

> to the Maior of Leicester & the Ald[e]r[m]en his brethren to acquainte them with his condic[i]on & to desire them to take a speedy course to convey him thither or to allow & pay some reasonable moneyes weekly towards the charge of his keeping in Bethlem[21]

the governors are both demanding that the parish meet its obligations, according to law, and also informing a community which might be ignorant of the condition of one of its members.

Obviously many parishes, public bodies and individuals used Bethlem more as a place of confinement than of cure. The hospital rarely questioned the motives of petitioners like Samuel Wilson who confessed to merely having regard to rid himself of a woman who was 'Troublesome att his do[ore],'[22] or Dr Richard Burd who, unconcerned with the cure of Margaret Hebb, 'was forced to get her into the said hosp[ita]ll' a second time because 'she had continued to vex and trouble the petic[i]oner in a most insupportable manner'.[23] Nevertheless, there is no doubting, that the hospital and the majority of petitioners were interested in the cure of the individuals concerned.[24] Governors were informed in their 'Charge' that the hospital was 'for cureing needy deplorable Lunaticks'.[25] Applicants ordinarily expressed this hope in their petitions, and the Court at Bethlem concurred by stressing cure as a standard objective in its admission orders.[26] Despite their respectful tone, the governors gave short shrift to Parliament's attempt to use the hospital as a prison or Bridewell in 1675, informing its Clerk that

John Taylor (committed for blasphemy) was not lunatic, nor was the hospital a place of punishment.[27] In the annual Spital reports the hospital boasted of its success in curing its patients and, by the later seventeenth century, touted figures advertising an average cure-rate of over two-thirds.[28] This was both by way of an appeal to the public for the continuance of their charity, and proof of its current efficacy. Dr Edward Tyson was praised and his annual gratuity increased by the governors for 'Curing a much greater number of the said Lunaticks . . . then ever had been proporc[i]onably cured in times foregoeing'.[29]

Although in practice chronic cases continued to silt up the hospital in the seventeenth and eighteenth centuries, the Admission Registers, commencing in 1683, reveal that the vast majority were short-stay cases, who remained for less than two, and increasingly for only one year, a fact seldom appreciated by historians. Patients were supposed to stay in Bethlem only as long as they remained in a condition that made it impossible to maintain them elsewhere. Thus patients were commonly discharged as able to 'bee kept in any other place as well as here'.[30] With the hospital constantly stretched to its capacity, the emphasis at Bethlem was increasingly on restricting space to the most 'needy', which encouraged speedy cure and a rapid turnover. Thus priorities of charity, in one respect, gave urgent impetus to those of therapy. While this meant that patients were often ejected before complete recovery, that considerations of security became pre-eminent in admission and discharge, and that cure was often only an estimate of how agreeable and tractable a patient might be in the hospital or community, this is not very different from the ethos governing many modern psychiatric institutions. Moreover, this policy of discharging patients while only convalescent was universal to contemporary hospitals, although in the eighteenth century administrators were criticized for discharging patients too soon.[31]

During the late seventeenth and early eighteenth centuries, the emphasis on cure at Bethlem was heightened by determined efforts to remove chronic cases deemed incurable from the hospital. Orders directing clear-outs of incurables, so that the hospital could receive those considered most 'in need of the Charity' of Bethlem, because 'capable of receiving their Cures therein',[32] eventually issued in 1708 in the devising of a standard procedure for their extirpation.[33] In addition, the Minutes of the Bethlem Sub-Committee manifest the rejection, in the first place, of a great many applicants designated beyond the curative competence of the hospital.[34] To be considered 'a proper Object for the Charity of this house' actually meant, not just to be considered lunatic and poor, but curable too. Thus, charity involved therapy. The almost coercive commitment of the hospital to cure in the eighteenth century is demonstrated by its policy of barring those patients from readmission whose families insisted on removing them, contrary to the opinion of the doctor and committee that they were unwell and unfit for discharge.[35] This is enough, on its own, to suggest how untenable are the efforts of historians to distinguish sharply between a charity and a hospital during this period.

Although Bethlem did expand its capacity so that, after 1728, it could cater for mounting numbers of incurables, even this provision can be interpreted as a product of the enhanced stress upon cure at the hospital, rather than as any cynical recognition of the limitations to the efficacy of its care.[36] No doubt the type of relief with which the hospital furnished incurables accords most comfortably with the exclusive concept of Bethlem as a charity for lunatics. Incurables were maintained with the customary material benefits which Bethlem had to offer, but were denied any strictly medical attention for their mental illness. The rationales of charity, which had identified incurables as objects of neglect and as threats to others or themselves, were paramount and exclusivist. However, Bethlem still ministered as a hospital to their physical ailments, as it did to all its patients, and moreover gave its physician a mandate to apply any medicaments he thought fit if an incurable showed signs of recovery.[37] The environment of the hospital was regarded as therapeutic in itself for both curables and incurables and the occasional recovery of incurables in the hospital could be agreeably incorporated into popular medical theories about the superior power of Nature over medicine in inveterate illnesses.

From the late seventeenth century, at least, Bethlem actively co-operated to stimulate the recovery of both categories of patient, by granting leaves of absence as aids to recovery. Benjamin Billingsley, for instance, was allowed a month's furlough in 'the Country' in 1682, 'to trye if the aire will doe him any good'.[38] The Admission Registers are increasingly full of such examples. Towards the end of the eighteenth century, over twenty patients every year were being granted leave,[39] although the majority of leave was allowed for bodily (as far as it could be distinguished from mental) illness or at the request of obligors themselves, rather than as part of the therapeutic policy of the hospital.

If Bethlem was behaving like an almshouse in distributing money and clothing to poor patients, it was also increasingly providing a primitive form of after-care, and cure was an integral constituent in this relief. Thus in 1683, Jane Deakin, a vagrant 'formerly taken wandring about the streetes', was both cured and given '20s. to supply her wants till she can provide for herselfe in some Service'.[40] This type of relief was not extended into any regular system, until Tyson left an annuity to Bethlem in 1708. Thereafter patients 'known to be very poor and unprovided for' received 'a sume of money not exceeding 40s. . . . towards their present subsistence or finding them clothes', to defray their expenses on their way home, or to give them a start towards getting 'a Livelihood'.[41] While this alms was not directly concerned with the cure of patients, it was only given to those who had been 'cured in the said hospital'.[42]

Of course, Bethlem's brand of charity had a liberal dose of rhetoric or propagandist puff about it. Cure frequently gave way to relapse, and the hospital records are replete with cases of readmission and of patients being 'cured' two or three times in the space of a few years (although such cases deserve a more comprehensive statistical analysis than is feasible here).[43] Nevertheless, the governors were neither unaware of, nor unresponsive to, the problem of relapse. Although little specific was done to combat relapse in the seventeenth century, patients like Anne Kingston might have their discharge deferred until they had completed a course of medicine, even if they had, to all appearances, recovered.[44] Bethlem throughout this period recognized a primary responsibility to its own cases, and gradually came to guarantee priority in admissions to those patients who had been discharged cured and who had subsequently relapsed.[45] In 1772 (by which time admissions were conducted according to a rigid rotational system and the waiting-list had grown to a prodigious length), the governors ordered that any incurable who relapsed, having been discharged well, should immediately be placed at the top of the list for readmission.[46] John Haslam, apothecary to Bethlem (1795–1815), maintained, in 1798, that 'the majority' of cases, 'where they relapse . . . are sent back to Bethlem'.[47] At the turn of the eighteenth century, moreover, the establishment of a facility for cured patients 'to procure themselves a little necessary Phisick at the Spring and fall of the yeare' (through Tyson's initiative and benefactions) was wholly concerned with after-care and the prevention of relapse. This was both 'consistant w[i]th the Charity of this hosp[ita]ll' and also with its therapeutic function, between which the governors rarely distinguished.[48] From this juncture, out-patients became an integral part of the medical relief Bethlem provided.[49] In addition, by the mid-eighteenth century patients certified as recovered by the physician were being retained in the hospital for up to an extra six weeks, to confirm that their restitution was authentic.[50]

Most of all, the impression of Bethlem as an unchanging institution, which stubbornly refused to adapt to the outside world, with a long line of physicians content merely to repeat traditional and increasingly out-moded treatments, needs to be tempered. There is no doubt that the array of bleedings, vomits, purges, and so on, criticized by mad-doctors like William Battie[51] and by ex-patients themselves, like James Carkesse and Alexander Cruden (who had both been in Bethlem),[52] remained relatively unaltered at the hospital. Yet these therapies had stayed generally in vogue for all kinds of illnesses besides insanity throughout the seventeenth and eighteenth centuries and retained considerable orthodoxy in the face of criticism. The oft-rehearsed account of uniform physicking at Bethlem in particular merits closer analysis when, even in the seventeenth century, Dr Thomas Allen was explicitly instructed by the governors on his appointment, to 'be careful to see and speake w[i]th every Lunatike before hee p[re]scribeth any physicke for him from tyme to tyme'.[53] Dosages were supposed to be adapted to a patient's constitution. That by the eighteenth century patients were regularly admitted on trial, at the doctor's discretion, to determine whether they were 'strong enough to undergo a Course of Physicke', and were discharged if subsequently found unable to do so, is proof enough of some form of ongoing assessment of medication.[54] Nor were the governors oblivious to the question of the quality (or even efficacy) of their medicaments. In 1750 the committees of both Bridewell and Bethlem, supplemented by the special expertise of the governors who were physicians or apothecaries, examined 'the Goodness of the Medicines Administered to the patients and whether any & what Alternatives are proper to be made'.[55] Indeed the committee included Battie himself, who gave no sign of dissenting from its report a month later that no 'bad Medicines have been Admin[i]stered to the Patients'.[56] The governors made further efforts to improve the administering of physic, at this juncture, by making the apothecary a full-time resident member of staff and by erecting an apothecary's shop (or dispensary) at the hospital.[57] That this shop was modelled on that at St Bartholomew's Hospital, and was fitted-up under the supervision of the medical staff and governor-apothecaries at Bethlem, is a clear indication that the hospital was not isolated from salutary initiatives outside its own walls, and also of the increasing influence that medical expertise was now exerting on its running.[58]

Neither the governors nor the medical staff at Bethlem were prepared *simply* to implement the same faithful remedies for 200 years. That post-mortems were conducted by practitioners at the hospital during both centuries, is a sure sign that they were active and interested in broadening their understanding of insanity. In the seventeenth century Thomas Allen and Edward Tyson both certainly conducted post-mortems upon Bethlem patients.[59] Indeed they may have utilized a room which was specifically being set aside at the completion of the new Moorfields building 'for Doct[or] Allen the Phisitian to open the Bodyes of Lunatickes'.[60] While I have unearthed no evidence, as yet, for the continuance of autopsies by the physicians of Bethlem, in the late eighteenth century its controversial apothecary, John Haslam, devoted an entire treatise to this subject based on his autopsies at Bethlem.[61]

Cold bathing had been introduced to Bethlem in the 1680s, apparently on the governors' own initiative (although possibly on Dr Tyson's advice), when this therapy was still very much the rage.[62] The caution of the governors, who were careful to advise with their physician and through committees over the cost of such new treatments, is an instructive pointer as to how far hospitals had to measure therapeutic innovation against expense at this time. Tyson was also consulted by Sir John Floyer before Floyer compiled his *History of Cold Bathing* of 1702, 'about curing Madness by Cold Baths', and informed him 'That he had used it successfully on a Woman who designed to drown herself'.[63] Clearly the Bethlem physician was not always so far behind contemporary therapeutics as historians have been led to believe. Bathing was still being practised at Bethlem in the latter half of the eighteenth century, by which time a facility for hot bathing had also been added.[64] At the end of this century, a shower bath was installed, to up-date water-therapy at the hospital on the suggestion and by the authority of Dr Thomas Monro, who regarded the provision as 'much for the benefit of the patients'.[65]

Only a year before, Monro had on the same grounds introduced electrical therapy to Bethlem at a cost of £7 7s.[66] Although this was four years after the Electrical Dispensary had been founded in London, and also post-dated the electrical department at St Thomas's Hospital, Monro had been interested in electrical therapy for some years, and sufficiently motivated to send one of his patients, with an established 'moping melancholy', to John Birch, surgeon at St Thomas's, 'for experiment'.[67]

Indeed despite (or because of) valid grounds for the traditional image of Bethlem physicians as arch-conservatives, uninterested in the study of insanity at Bethlem, clear signs of their dedication and concern for patients' health, as manifested in the Court and Committee Minutes of the hospital, have received little attention. Whatever the evidence of the 1815–16 parliamentary inquiry,[68] these minutes reveal how (in accordance with their part-time contracts) physicians normally attended the hospital at least once, and often twice a week. Thomas Monro, badly implicated by the inquiry, emerges from these minutes as in many respects a model hospital physician. For example, he volunteered in 1793 that the position of new beds was likely to precipitate accidents to patients;[69] a week later, he recommended, along with Bryan Crowther, the surgeon (1789–1815), that improvements might be made to the patients' clothing, 'more conducive to their health and Cleanliness';[70] in 1794 he examined and advised on two rooms 'for the use of convalescent patients';[71] he testified in 1796 that the state of the privies was a great hazard to the patients' health;[72] he repeatedly advised on dietary changes and on the merits of the diet as it stood;[73] and he testified in 1800 to the insalubrity of patients being crowded together 'two in a Cell'[74] (a practice which seems to have been the exception rather than the rule at Bethlem). Earlier in the period, Tyson's reforms are well known, and while historians know little about Richard Hale, he was praised by his contemporaries, in Harveian Oration after Oration, for his successful and sympathetic treatment of the insane.[75] The physicians of the hospital were generally acknowledged by contemporaries as experts in their field.

Even in the seventeenth century, the governors of Bethlem recognized the remedial potential of management and strove to segregate the population of the hospital along very basic therapeutic lines. With the addition of twenty cells in the 1640s, those considered the 'most quiet & orderly' were isolated from 'the most outragious' in a separate wing.[76] While visitors commented on the lack of discrimination between the violent and pacific patients in Moorfields, patients were accorded the freedom of the house in the eighteenth century (i.e. permitted to walk in the Galleries) only if they were well-behaved. Alexander Cruden actually commended the system at Bethlem whereby patients were deprived of their privileges and subjected to restraint only if they were unruly.[77] Those patients found 'low Spirited or Inclinable to be Mopish' were, on the other hand, supposed to be 'obliged to get up' and 'Turned out of their Cells, [and] the Doors Locked, that they may not creep back again to their Beds'.[78] Despite the draconian tone of this type of management, which required servants to 'Acquaint the Physician when ever any of the patients (without particular Sickness) take to their Beds' and to 'Employ such of the Patients at their Needle as are Capable when not otherwise busied rather than Let them Walk Idle up and down the House Shewing it to Strangers and begging Money',[79] this is not so far removed as we have come to expect from the popular moral therapy of the later eighteenth century.[80] While such directives commonly represent ideals rather than practice, or expedients rather than a philosophy, historians need familiarizing with these ideals. Moreover, within the context of the eighteenth-century association of insanity with idleness, the governors of Bethlem appear to have been thoroughly *au fait* with current therapeutics. We might even regard them as reaching towards a more progressive or modern form of occupational therapy. In 1779 the patients were provided with two sets of skittles.[81] Throughout the period under consideration, there are instances of tractable or convalescent patients being employed and paid as helpers in the hospital, although less indeed with a mind to their recovery than to ease the extreme problems of under-staffing which beset most contemporary hospitals.[82]

Historians are already familiar with some of the shortcomings of Bethlem as a medical centre. In an attempt to restore a balance, this chapter has given an extremely incomplete account of charity and therapeutics at the hospital. Yet I have also omitted many other details of Bethlem's provision, particularly environmental aspects like diet, air and hygiene, which were crucial to its functioning as a hospital. Moreover, the continual and improving attention of Bethlem to the bodily health of its patients (by, for example, the appointment of a nurse, in the seventeenth century, or the establishment of infirmaries in the mid-eighteenth century)[83] is a subject I have barely touched on, and an obvious sphere in which the charity of Bethlem was concerned with medical treatment. Nor is it entirely true to say that the hospital was solely for 'pauper' lunatics.[84]

Ultimately the governors still seem to have been more concerned with extending the spatial boundaries of their charity by continually adding more cells, than with radically altering the type of therapy practised therein. Bethlem remained very much an institution for the poor, and as such was usually a poorer alternative to private care offered elsewhere. As late as 1790, the fears of relatives like John Luskin who, upon a vacancy arising for his allegedly incurable mother on the Bethlem establishment, preferred to keep her in the care of 'a very Creditable family', give one very valid view of the inferior care Bethlem appeared to provide. Despite the 'very heavy Expence', Luskin and his family were assured in the knowledge that she would be treated with 'kindness' and 'indulgence', and that she was only 'half a mile' away and could be seen 'as often as we please'. By sending her to Bethlem, they would have been forced 'to part from her, and perhaps never see her more'.[85] However, other relatives, even those who had tried alternative means first, turned to Bethlem with genuine hopes of alleviation. That notorious courtesan, Teresia Constantia Phillips, related the (not implausible) story of a surgeon's daughter, who, having 'continued for above three Years' at 'a private Madhouse', 'was given over by all the Physicians as incurable'. In sending her subsequently to Bethlem her parents not only believed that 'the Expence of her Maintenance would . . . be lessened' but also had 'Hopes of her still being relieved, by the different Methods of treating her'. Sure enough, partly through the sensitivity and vigilance of the staff, she recovered.[86]

The charity of Bethlem provided both alms and medical treatment, both care and cure, and accepted both public and private cases. Historians, who have sought to delineate the 'birth of the hospital' in the genesis of modern diagnostics, therapeutics and professional structures, have applied an anachronistic methodology to early modern institutions, derided the inclusiveness of early modern charity, and erroneously presupposed a contradiction in terms between 'a hospital [and] a charity'. This is not to deny, of course, that there were areas of fundamental conflict between the priorities of fund-raising publicity (in the widest sense) and material succour, and those of therapy. Bethlem has long been of paradigmatic value for historians. We must now begin to appreciate the many other dimensions to the paradigm of Bethlem, beyond the polarities in which its history has been locked.

NOTES

1 R. Hunter and I. Macalpine, *Three Hundred Years of Psychiatry, 1535–1860*, Oxford, 1963, p. 199 (though cf. ibid., p. 105).

2 For this view and its refutation, see Hunter and Macalpine, op. cit., passim; A. T. Scull, *Museums of Madness*, London, 1979, esp. pp. 54, 63, 74–5; Scull (ed.) *Mad-Houses, Mad-Doctors and Madmen: The Social History of Psychiatry in the Victorian Era*, London, 1981; P. H. Allderidge, 'Bedlam: fact or fantasy', in W. F. Bynum, R. Porter and M. Shepherd (eds) *The Anatomy of Madness: Essays in the History of Psychiatry*, 2 vols, London, 1985, vol. 2, pp. 17–33; and J. Andrews, 'The lot of the "incurably" insane in Enlightenment England', *Eighteenth-Century Life*, 1988, vol. 12.

3 See for example the Bethlem Court of Governors Minutes (henceforth BCGM), 19 December 1708, when its wording was slightly altered.

4 That is Bridewell (which had the same board of governors as Bethlem), St Thomas's, St Bartholomew's and Christ's. Most charitable foundations during this period advertised by means of annual sermons.

5 The Spital sermons were preached every Easter at the church of St Mary Spittal until the Restoration and thereafter at St Bridget's. They seem to have begun during the Civil War, but Bethlem was not included as part of their agenda until 1644 (see BCGM, 15 March, 4 and 17 April 1644 and 2 April 1645). They were printed under the title, *A Sermon Preach'd before the Right-Honourable The Lord-Mayor, Aldermen and Governours of the Several Hospitals of the City of London*. From the 1680s at least, they contained reports, with statistics, on the state of the hospitals as also in the years 1645–56, when they were entitled *A True Report of the Great Costs and Charges of the Five Hospitals in the City of London*, or sometimes found under the title, *A Psalm of Thanksgiving to be Sung by the Children of Christ's Hospital, on Monday, Tuesday and Wednesday in Easter Week, according to Ancient Custom, for their Founders and Benefactors*. Sermons and reports served generally as a means of fund-raising for both the ordinary running of the hospitals and occasionally for more specific purposes such as the extension of Bethlem's incurable wards: see for example James Ibbetson's Spital sermon, *The Case of Incurable Lunaticks and the Charity due to them particularly recommended*, London, 1759.

6 See Bethlem certificate in BCGM, 2 April 1645, for example. Treasurers and auditors were not always able to keep their accounts in the black (ibid., 12 May and 28 July 1641; and E. G. O'Donoghue, *The Story of Bethlehem Hospital*, London, 1914, pp. 166, 179).

7 See BCGM, 11 April 1701, 6 November 1702, 18 July 1738, 16 July 1789 and Bethlem Grand Committee Minutes (henceforth BGCM) 11 July 1789.

8 For Moorfields, see BCGM, 19 May, 16 July and 10 September 1675. By the middle of the eighteenth century, nearly £9,000 in donations and assets had been pledged exclusively to the relief of incurables in Bethlem. See Andrews, op. cit., p. 5. Yet for borrowing by the governors, see

BCGM, 12 July 1728 and 5 April 1737.

9 The foundations of St Luke's, the Westminster Infirmary and the Lock Hospital, for example.

10 BCGM, 9 September 1641.

11 BCGM, 23 October 1674; cf. BCGM, 5 May 1676.

12 See the extract from the Registry of the Prerogative Court in Box 65, archives of the Royal Bethlem Hospital. The will was dated 8 September 1798, and proved on 12 September.

13 BCGM and Bethlem Sub-Committee Minutes (henceforth BSCM).

14 Indeed the earliest instance of its usage I have found in the records does not occur until 1692 (BCGM, 29 July 1692).

15 By 'obligors', I mean those who entered into bonds or obtained bondsmen for the support of patients in Bethlem.

16 BCGM, 6 August 1656 (case of Mary Wilkinson).

17 Ibid., 28 October 1653.

18 Ibid., 7 February 1655. Cf. M. Foucault, *Folie et déraison: Histoire de la folie à l'âge classique*, Paris, 1961, for which see the English abridged translation, *Madness and Civilisation: A History of Insanity in the Age of Reason*, London, 1965, esp. ch. 2.

19 BCGM, 24 September 1651.

20 Individuals acting as guardians for their insane relatives might be 'induced' to support them in Bethlem for as long as they could afford to do so, and 'to go into service' and penury in order to continue the weekly payments, like the mother and sister of Margaret Hebb in 1696: BCGM, 16 December 1696.

21 BCGM, 31 March 1652.

22 BCGM, 13 January 1656.

23 BCGM, 12 February 1697.

24 For a vindication of the reality of Bethlem as a centre of cure, see Allderidge, op. cit.

25 BCGM, 19 December 1707.

26 BCGM. Petitions for admission to Bethlem seem to survive only from the eighteenth century (see Box 'D' in the Bethlem archives), but the admissions orders in the Court of Governors' Minutes are clearly paraphrasing petitions.

27 BCGM, 19 May 1675, and transcript of letter from John Browne, Clerk of Parliament, dated 14 May 1675, at the back of the same Court Book.

28 See note 4; John Strype's edition of John Stowe's *A Survey of the Cities of London and Westminster*, London, 1720, pp. 192–7; and Hunter and Macalpine, op. cit., p. 308.

29 BCGM, 12 October 1694.

30 BCGM.

31 For example at St Thomas's Hospital, which is partly what prompted Thomas Guy to found his own hospital in 1721. See H. C. Cameron, *Mr Guy's Hospital*, London, 1954, pp. 26, 41, 45–6.

32 BCGM, 1 July and 17 August 1681; 11 April 1701; and 6 November 1702; and also Admissions Registers around 1701–2.

33 BCGM, 14 May 1708.

34 Between 1708 and 1728 seventy-seven patients were recorded as rejected

for being: too weak to undergo a course of physic; too old or infirm; sane or 'pretty well'; epileptic, convulsive or mopish; already discharged as incurable or because of the inveteracy of their illnesses, etc. (BSCM). I assume that a great many more rejections went unrecorded.

35 See for example BSCM, 7 October 1710, 10 January 1719, 8 September and 13 October 1764. On the other hand, see too 29 June and 3 August 1765, 26 July and 29 August 1767, 16 December 1768 and 3 June 1769, when there is no record of patients removed against the consent of the committee being barred.

36 For further discussion on this point, see Andrews, op. cit.

37 See 'Incurables – Rules for Governm[en]t of ye Patients &c', 4th and 7th rules, BCGM, 12 July 1728.

38 BCGM, 16 June 1682.

39 See the Discharge Register for 1782–1810, for example, where the furloughs of forty-two men and forty-seven women are recorded between February 1782 and September 1785.

40 BCGM, 7 September 1683.

41 BCGM, 3 September 1708 (abstract of Tyson's will) and BSCM.

42 BCGM.

43 John Haslam, apothecary to Bethlem (1795–1816), calculated that over 13 per cent of those patients admitted during 1796 and 1797 were readmissions: Haslam, *Observations on Insanity: with Practical Remarks on the Disease, and an Account of the Morbid Appearances on Dissection*, London, 1798, p. 109.

44 BCGM, 18 November 1681.

45 See the readmission of Anne Smith in 1673, however, which was justified by considerations of security rather than therapy: BCGM, 23 April 1673. Plainly it was the concept of a threat, whether personal or social, which dictated the readmission of relapsed patients at Bethlem.

46 BSCM, 22 February 1772. This regulation may, however, have been belatedly modelled on the admissions policy at St Luke's Hospital, which guaranteed priority to those patients who had relapsed within two months of their discharge (St Luke's Sub-Committee Minutes). Moreover, preferential admission for relapsed 'ex-incurables' seems to have been rescinded at Bethlem in 1785 (BSCM, 26 February and 5 March 1785 and 10 February 1787).

47 Haslam, op. cit., p. 109.

48 BCGM, 26 April 1700; cf. Tyson's will referred to at note 41.

49 In 1718 John Wheeler, surgeon to Bethlem (1714–40), supported by Richard Hale, the physician (1708–28), claimed to have 'annually blooded ab[ou]t a thousand in & out patients belonging to both hospitals' (BCGM, 10 January and 14 February 1718).

50 See T. S. Phillips, *An Apology for the Conduct of Mrs T. C. .*, London, 1759, vol. 3, pp. 88–9.

51 W. Battie, *A Treatise on Madness* (1758), ed. R. Hunter and I. Macalpine, London, 1962.

52 J. Carkesse, *Lucida Intervalla: Containing Divers Miscellaneous Poems*, London, 1679; and A. Cruden, *The Adventures of Alexander the Corrector*, London, 1754, who called these remedies 'The common

Prescriptions of a Bethlematical Doctor' and 'no great Mystery', p. 24. See also Cruden's *Mr Cruden Greatly Injured*, London, 1739, pp. 29–30. Cruden was admitted to Bethlem on 17 December 1743 and then discharged on 3 March 1744. See Bethlem Admissions Register fol. 184.

53 BCGM, 26 June 1667.
54 See for example BSCM, 23 June 1711, 10 May 1718, 17 January 1719, 27 January 1723 and 1 November 1729.
55 BCGM, 12 April 1750.
56 BCGM, 16 May 1750. Although the administration of Bethlem may have been more concerned with the *quality* of medicaments than their *efficacy*, these concerns were not unconnected. The establishment of the apothecary's shop in the hospital at this stage suggests that the governors were increasingly concerned about their suppliers.
57 The apothecary was henceforth to attend daily, Monday to Saturday, instead of just three times per week. See BCGM, 1 February 1751, and BSCM, 17 February 1751. The Grand Committee initially – mysteriously – rejected the proposal for a resident apothecary (BSCM, 5 December 1750), but the Court of Governors overruled it on this (BSCM, 14 December 1750, and BCGM, 27 April 1769).
58 BCGM, 16 May 1750.
59 See R. Wiseman, *Several Chirurgical Treatises*, London, 1676, vol. 1, p. 132; Hunter and Macalpine, op. cit., pp. 227–9; and T. Birch, *The History of the Royal Society of London*, London, 1756, vol. 3, p. 502 (17 November 1756).
60 BCGM, 12 January 1676.
61 Haslam, op. cit.
62 For bathing at Bethlem, see BCGM, 7 July 1687, 29 June 1688, 24 May and 28 June 1689; BSCM, 13 May 1710 (when ten 'Bathing frocks' are provided for the hospital); 19 and 26 March 1757 (when repairs are ordered to the women's cold bath); and BGCM, 24 March 1795 (when a 'Bathing Jacket' is purchased). For water therapy generally, see E. Baynard and J. Floyer, *The History of Cold Bathing Both Ancient and Modern in Two Parts*, London, 1702; Floyer, *An Enquiry into the Right Use and Abuses of the Hot, Cold and Temperate Baths in England*, London, 1697; F. M. von Helmont, *The Spirit of Disease*, London, 1692; R. Pierce, *Bath Memoirs*, Bristol, 1697; and Hunter and Macalpine, op. cit., pp. 123, 254–7, 268–70, 325–9.
63 Baynard and Floyer, op. cit., p. 142.
64 BSCM, 7 February 1778.
65 BSCM, 20 January 1798; BGCM, 23 February and 31 July 1798. The innovation cost only £1 15s. The douche continued to be widely deployed in nineteenth-century asylums.
66 BSCM, 24 December 1796; BGCM, 3 February 1797.
67 See J. Birch, *A Letter to the Author*, in G. Adams, *An Essay on Electricity*, London, 1792, pp. 565–6; and Hunter and Macalpine, op. cit., pp. 534–61.
68 *Report[s] from the [Select] Committee on Madhouses in England*, London, 1815–16, first and fourth reports, esp. pp. 35, 92.

69 BSCM, 9 November 1793.
70 BSCM, 16 November 1793.
71 BGCM, 6 May 1794.
72 BGCM, 20 August 1796.
73 BGCM, 9 July 1795; BSCM, 19 March 1796.
74 BSCM, 7 June 1800.
75 See for example *Harveian Orations* of Pierce Dod (1729), pp. 14–15; of J. Hollings (1734), pp. 46–7; of Edward Wilmot (1735), pp. 17–18; and of James Munro (1737), pp. 22–3, in the Library of the Royal College of Physicians, London. See also J. Andrews, 'A respectable mad-doctor? Richard Hale FRS', *Notes and Records of the Royal Society of London*, 1990, vol. 44.
76 Even if the governors seem to have been as much concerned with the disturbance of their tenants as with their patients: BCGM, 21 July 1645 and 21 January 1663.
77 Cruden, 1754, op. cit., p. 13.
78 BCGM, 20 June 1765, Memorial of Grand Committee, dated 19 June.
79 Ibid.
80 Haslam, op. cit., pp. 127–9 (withholding privileges from patients); A. Digby, 'Moral treatment at the York Retreat', in Bynum, Porter and Shepherd, op. cit.; and Digby, *Madness, Morality and Medicine. A Study of the York Retreat, 1796–1914*, Cambridge, 1985.
81 BSCM, 17 July 1779.
82 Although this is a complex issue which cannot be properly dealt with here, there seems little sign that employment of patients was viewed as part of therapy.
83 BCGM, 16 December 1692; 13 and 27 January 1693; 15 March 1700; 30 July and 9 September 1741; 17 February and 12 March 1742; and 8 August 1753; BSCM, 24 August 1753.
84 A large number of patients were supported by their families, not the poor rate. While patients were increasingly excluded from the hospital if they were found to have means enough to be supported elsewhere, Bethlem also increasingly discriminated against parish patients. Some patients were described as ladies or gentlemen: for example BCGM, 16 August 1637, 3 January and 28 February 1638, 21 April 1648, 30 June 1671, 17 November 1676; BSCM, 22 December 1716.
85 BGCM, 28 August 1790. For isolation, even from family and visitors, see BSCM, 22 January, 28 May 1785, 6 May 1797 and 1815–16 Commons Enquiry on James Tilly Matthews.
86 Phillips, op. cit., vol. 3, pp. 71–2.

5

TWO MEDICAL CHARITIES IN EIGHTEENTH-CENTURY LONDON

The Lock Hospital and the Lying-In Charity for Married Women

Donna Andrew

Eighteenth-century men and women congratulated themselves on their charitableness. They had just reason for pride. In the thirty years between 1740 and 1770 at least two dozen charities of miscellaneous sorts were founded in London and supported by concerned groups of private citizens, pooling their resources and contributing their time and effort to the management and direction of voluntary poor relief.[1] Many of these charities took as their goal the treatment of a variety of medical conditions and problems. In this way the history of London's eighteenth-century charities is intimately interwoven with the history of medicine in eighteenth-century London, of which we still know little, and need to know much more.

In this chapter I should like to look at two of these medical, charitable institutions in greater detail, examining their origins, their purposes, the sorts of people they attracted as donors and governors, and their successes and failures. These are the Lying-in Charity and the Lock Hospital. Because both dealt with medical conditions resulting from sexual contact, the history of both reflects, among other things, contemporary opinions about sexuality. And because both appealed for funds and managers to a similar group of potential donors, we can compare and contrast them.

First, a word must be said about sources. Charities in the eighteenth century used a variety of approaches to disseminate appeals and solicit funds. Newspaper advertisements, charity dinners

82

and benefit concerts were employed to draw attention to the hopes and aspirations, as well as the day-to-day operations of these institutions. Many institutions also printed yearly 'declarations of purpose' to convince old donors to give again, and new donors to begin. For all these societies depended upon annual and life subscriptions for the bulk of their income.[2] One of the most popular methods of persuading people to be charitable was the annual charity sermon. These sermons were attempts to convince their audiences of the efficacy of their particular charity, and of its national social or policy value. Thus the charity sermons speak to us in voices louder than their own, for in many ways they articulated the hopes and motives of their audiences whose opinions otherwise are almost entirely unknown and unrecorded.

In addition to humanitarian and Christian motives to charity, a host of others undoubtedly operated as well. As early as the 1730s, that cynical physician, Bernard Mandeville, noted that people gave to charity for various non-altruistic reasons, to be able to dominate the poor and to find themselves in the company of the rich. Others wished for praise, he said, for salvation, or to relieve the uneasiness the sight of the distressed occasioned. 'Pride and Vanity', he wrote, 'have built more Hospitals than all other [Christian] Virtues together.'[3] It is clear, however, that even if donors to hospitals hoped more for spiritual than for solid financial rewards, as Mandeville had claimed, the sight of one's name underneath that of an aristocrat, an MP or a City magnate on a subscription list must have been both gratifying and financially useful. These subscription lists are another source of information of who gave, and in what amount. Finally, for the Lock Hospital, a most valuable but curiously underused source remains – the minutes of the committee meetings and deliberations of the boards of direction themselves.[4]

Before we can understand the novelty of the first society we shall examine, the Lying-in Charity for Delivering Poor Married Women in their Own Habitations (henceforth the Lying-in Charity), we must consider what had already been done to provide charitable assistance in childbirth to poor and needy women before it even began.

The notion that the state or community should aid poor pregnant women was not very new. Both Sir William Petty and Mandeville thought the state should make itself responsible for safer and hence more scientific childbirth in the interests of the nation.[5] In practice, however, little had been done. Although Sir Richard Manningham, an early practitioner and teacher of obstetrics, had opened a ward for lying-in women in the parochial infirmary of St James's, Westminster, in 1739, and the Middlesex opened a similar ward in 1747, the British Lying-in Hospital for Poor Married Women was the first specialized institution dealing only in the delivery of children in London. This hospital, founded in 1740, and those that followed it owed their start, in some part, to an increasing interest in a scientific understanding of the birth process. In addition to the rash of technical manuals which appeared, and the growing use of obstetrical instruments, both Manningham and Smellie gave classes in obstetrics to the large number of male midwives wanting to enter this practice. There were those, however, who considered male interest in this field to be scandalous and improper. Many thought that childbirth should be returned to the sole charge of the female midwife.[6] In addition to charges of impropriety, there was a wider debate going on between the relative value of female midwives versus 'accoucheurs', as the male obstetricians liked to be called. There is no doubt that the hospitals benefited from the support and patronage given to them by the 'childbirth professionals', by the many concerned and famous surgeons, physicians and apothecaries who subscribed and worked for them.[7] Still, it seems fairly clear that this contest, and the public attention it aroused, were not the only, and probably not even the greatest reason for the foundation of these hospitals. In one of them at least, the training aspect was discounted;[8] furthermore most babies born in these hospitals were delivered without instruments by female midwives.[9] It is equally clear, however, that access to a great number of women in labour, and the opportunity to try out new modes of care for post-delivery difficulties, made these hospitals attractive to doctors and worthy of their support. The clearest case of this is in the career of Dr John Leake, founder in 1767 of the General Lying-in Hospital in Lambeth. Leake, having started medical practice on the survivors of the great Lisbon earthquake in 1755, got his degree at Rheims in 1763 and came to London determined to make his fortune. In his hospital Leake gave lessons in midwifery, invented a three-armed forceps, and practised rather strange experiments to stop haemorrhaging in post-partum women.[10] However, while it is quite clear that many doctors, especially those like Leake who had not had the capital to train in the more orthodox fashion, were attracted to this new area of care, this does not explain why the public supported, nay handsomely supported, the doctors in this interest. Why did Londoners of the mid-century decide that lying-in was a problem worthy of their concern?

One possible reason was the growth of a kind of sentimentalism at mid-century, exemplified perhaps in that forgotten bestseller, Mackenzie's *The Man of Feeling*. Thus the theme of the pregnant woman in danger of death was ripe with possibilities for eliciting charitable donations. This picture appealed to the sentiments, touched the heart, and aroused a desire to relieve the anguish of those who bestow life.[11] In addition, there were many pragmatic reasons for supporting a safer childbirth that must have appealed to the merchants and financiers who contributed to these institutions. Not only was it thought to be the obligation of the well-to-do to provide for the deserving poor in such times of need, but also the provision of lying-in aid was seen to be particularly useful in promoting hard work among this vitally important element in society. Women helped through their 'greatest exigencies [which will] redouble their labour, will work more cheerfully, and return to labour with better health'.[12] Not only industry, but also religion, would be promoted by such assistance, for women were provided with Bibles and visited regularly by clergymen who exhorted them to prayer and reflection. Children born in the hospitals were baptized in the attached chapels, and were thus started off as proper Christians. At least one lying-in hospital also demanded a public show of gratitude from women whom they had delivered, and threatened exclusion from further benefits if this was not forthcoming.[13]

Finally the hospitals claimed that while increasing and improving public morality through the promotion and reward of marriage, they were also aiding in the increase of England's numbers by the successful delivery of more babies, as well as by the conservation of many women as future productive and reproductive citizens. For with few exceptions most of the lying-in hospitals would aid only poor *married* women, and often demanded written proof of this status before care was forthcoming. Both the British and the City of London Lying-in Hospitals made it quite clear that they were in no way encouraging licentiousness, that the women they were treating were truly deserving, and that their institutions were examples of

> an open testimony borne in favour of the first ordinance of Heaven [i.e. marriage]; on which not only the comfort, but the very support of human life so greatly depends; which is the foundation of families and government.[14]

It was the avowed and often repeated purpose of these institutions to strengthen marriage, families and government. In so far as marriage was seen as being most conducive to population growth, and that in turn to the expansion of commerce and empire, these institutions served primarily national purposes. The grand aspirations of these hospitals is well illustrated by the following excerpt from a Prologue read for the benefit of the City of London Lying-in Hospital:

> Each hardy son, whom this night's alms shall raise,
> Will to Great Britain consecrate his days;
> Her arts, her commerce, her domain extend,
> Or force her haughty enemies to bend;
> Whilst the fair daughters of this genial day
> Shall serve their country – in a gentler way;
> If doom'd as humble spinsters to grow old,
> Shall spin our envy'd fleeces into gold;
> If wedded, shall with Hymen's magic chain
> From foreign climes our artizans refrain,
> From foreign climes recall the wandering tar,
> With hearts of oak supply the wastes of war
> And with sons' sons enrich our future store,
> Till time, and this great empire, are no more.[15]

Wishing a strong, wealthy state of many employed and virtuous citizens, contemporaries recognized that the source of such national wealth and power lay in labour and the labourer. The productivity of the labouring poor was the great motive force that kept the state healthy and strong. People, and especially labouring people, were seen to have a concrete *value*, quite distinct from their spiritual or intellectual worth. Labourers were often discussed as units of production, as 'hands' and their value measured in monetary terms. Lawrence Braddon, solicitor to the wine excise board, calculated that every 'poor young child . . . as soon as born, and likely to live, upon a political account, may be valued at £15'. Braddon added that these children, 'when well bred up, may be made the greatest wealth and strength of the nation'.[16] For population growth was seen as a cause of both national strength and national prosperity. The more people a nation had, the more formidable she would be in both war and peace. A large population was necessary to maintain international power, to man the fleet and armed forces, and to act as a bulwark against foreign depredations. So evident was the connection between numbers and power to social theorists, that *how* and not *why* population should increase became the problem tackled in pamphlets with titles like *An*

Essay or a Modest Proposal of a Way to Encrease the Number of People and Consequently the Strength of the Kingdom (1693).[17]

We have already noted Braddon's assessment of the value of every well-trained child as £15 per annum to the nation. Clearly the more units there were that could be multiplied by fifteen, the larger would be the national product. In addition to the direct value of the labour of a growing population, there would be beneficial side-effects. Through more intensive cultivation of land, an expansion of trade under the pressure of necessity and the consequent fall in wages of labour, the citizenry, 'to compensate for the diminution of their immediate profit, must study every method to render trade more certain and extensive than before'.[18] With the outbreak of the Seven Years War, and the destruction of population that the war would bring, it became even more important to aid women in childbirth, saving both maternal and infant lives for the service of the nation.

It was with the needs of the nation in mind that the Lying-in Charity was established in 1758. The proponents of this new form of lying-in care claimed that it could realize the goal of the hospitals, that is a safer and more painless childbirth, while eliminating the dangers that the hospitals invited of an over-generous or misplaced charity. The Lying-in Charity served the same sort of women as the hospitals, that is women who were married but too poor to afford private aid in childbirth. It proposed to send out midwives, as well as to lend linen, to women who had their babies at home. A doctor, the public was assured, was always standing by if needed, but in most cases a midwife could do the job as adequately, and far more cheaply. Not only did the charity show that it was doing more good for less money than the hospitals, but also it claimed that home delivery was safer than hospital confinement. Certainly the writings of medical men familiar with the hospitals suggest that they were unhealthy places. Little, if anything, was known about antiseptics, the causes of childbirth fevers, or the necessity to separate the ill and the well in such cases. In some of the lying-in hospitals the patients shared beds, and this no doubt encouraged the rapid spread of disease.[19] Furthermore, unlike the hospitals which allowed mothers about a month in bed, the charity claimed that it would, by delivering the women at home, force the husband to continue his efforts for her support. Thus, in contrast to the misdirected charity of the hospitals, the aid offered by the Lying-in Charity would be genuine, for while it reconciled 'Man to a Life of Labour, without removing the Necessity of it', its effects 'would redound equally to the advantage of himself and the Public'.[20]

In addition to the added bonus of paternal labour, the charity also noted the advantage of the woman's speedier return to productive labour. Unlike the long stay in bed common in the hospitals, a woman delivered at home

> at the End of Ten Days or a Fortnight . . . is able to manage her usual Business. [H]ere is the Advantage of so much Industry to the Public, and likewise a greater Service done to her Family.[21]

Finally, the delivery of women in their own homes would have an important and lasting influence on their families. For their uninterrupted presence at home was absolutely essential for family stability. It was the mother who was the guardian of family morals, whose watchful eye kept her husband working and her daughters chaste. Her lying-in, if at home, could be a splendid occasion for the exercise of practical morality. Her children, instead of forgetting the obedience they owed, instead of

> being left to themselves for several weeks, without the authority and direction of their parents . . . shall here be practiced in an essential duty, to comfort and assist those parents in distress. . . . Surely, there is an ingenious economy in this charity, that whilst infants are trained to virtue, their virtues are turned to good account.[22]

Promising all the advantages of a growing labour force at this time of national crisis, it is perhaps not surprising that the supporters of this new charity should have been overwhelmingly of the merchant class. Fewer than 2 per cent of them were aristocrats, for example. Though unusually supportive and active (two-thirds of the annual subscribers in 1767 were still present and active in 1770) they seem to have been cautious people, desiring to remain annual contributors.[23] By giving their support on a yearly basis they could keep a check on the operations of the charity, whereas if they had donated a large sum initially, they would have lost some of this control. While many members of the charity were undoubtedly of a deeply religious though tolerant bent (as witnessed by the substantial number of subscribers who also belonged to the Society for Promoting Christian Knowledge among the Poor –

an organization that distributed the works of middle-of-the-road theologians of *all* the Protestant denominations) it is unlikely that they were motivated by 'rapturous flights or wild chimeras'. Their frame of mind might best be described as 'rational and pious'. Their religion was sensible and their business interests were well entrenched. Many of them held offices in their guilds, acted as secretaries and lawyers to the large City companies or served on the boards of the City's growing number of insurance companies. In politics they seem to have been moderate and conservative; many were opposed to the 1769 Wilkes movement.[24] They appear to have been people who felt the obligations of Christian charity, but thought that prudence and public utility should dictate the direction of their contributions. In the Lying-in Charity they found an ideal vehicle for the most secure fulfilment of this obligation.

In many ways the Lying-in Charity subscribers represent the perfect sort of charitable donor. Though the charity was not enormous in numbers (by 1767 the charity had 381 subscribers), it had those sorts of contributors who had both the business acumen and the commercial and charity 'connections' to make a success of a new venture. Both Benjamin Barnett and his banking partner John Bland were donors. Robert Willson, a stationer and common councillor, as well as two other members of his family contributed. Frederick Pigou, director of the Sun Fire Office and an East India director and merchant, and Charles Green Say, printer of the *Daily Gazetteer*, also gave. By convincing such men to support the venture, the society assured itself of both good management and ongoing financial support.[25]

An interesting contrast to the success story of the Lying-in Charity is the history of the Lock Hospital. The Lock Hospital for the treatment and cure of venereal disease, established in 1746, met an obvious need, that is the widespread and growing incidence of such disorders in mid-century London. Almost every one has read of Boswell's many bouts with 'the pox' and his resort to mercury treatments. In fact venereal cures were one of the fastest growing and probably most lucrative of all the popular or quack cures on the London market. A very perfunctory glance at the advertisements in the London papers for the four months of May to August 1781 revealed at least six different promised cures, each with its own claims to efficacy. These remedies, available at booksellers, perfumers, toyshops, by mail or from the concocter personally, cost between 2s. 6d. and 5s. a box or bottle. Yet despite the obvious need for a public institution to treat those who could not have afforded such medication, the charity had great difficulty in convincing the public of the necessity of its existence. For there was a widespread belief that since, on the whole, venereal diseases proceeded naturally from sexual promiscuity, it would be wrong to alleviate well-deserved punishment. This kind of aid, it was feared, by making venereal disease less dangerous, would lead to an increase in sexual impropriety. Yet there were good, economic reasons to fear the effects of venereal disease on the nation. Although the evidence is lacking, it seems likely that the increased military and naval activity in this period served to spread and intensify the effects of these diseases. London must have been especially hard hit, since she was not only the depot for soldiers and sailors, but also the home base of a large maritime fleet. These men would have been the perfect subjects for, and carriers of, all sorts of venereal infections. Although the causes and treatment of such diseases were much misunderstood, it was known that people afflicted with these diseases were often unable to bear or engender children. The spread of these diseases, then, hindered that procreation which seemed so necessary from a national point of view. Not only did it take its toll in the ill-health of its victims and have national consequences in the reduction of the population, but also it ruined the health and lives of many innocent children and potentially useful citizens.[26]

Despite such appeals, however, the Lock Hospital tottered unsteadily through its first thirty years. While numbers cared for increased, the Lock faced continual problems of directorial support. Thirteen board meetings in these decades had to be cancelled because of insufficient attendance. In 1758, 1761 and 1762 subscriptions were much in arrears and tradesmen's bills unpaid. In May 1752 the governors had hired a collector in an attempt to bring in more of the promised donations; by January 1754 the governors were bringing an action against this very collector for retaining donated funds. The matron and the cook of the hospital were dismissed in May 1763 for not giving the patients their full food rations. By April 1765 the charity owed its tradesmen more than £1,100. Its survival during these decades seems to have been due to inadvertence and good fortune more than to planning and foresight.[27] For unlike the Lying-in, the Lock appealed almost entirely only to humane altruism and Christian sentiment. This, for example, is an excerpt from one of its sermons:

But if any notwithstanding, should say, what too many have said, that no Hospital should be supported, which is to relieve persons who willfully bring a disease upon themselves, through their own wickedness and abandoned life. To this I answer, 1st. It bespeaks a far better sense of our love of our neighbour, to be finding reasons for doing him good, than inventing, or even admitting excuses for withholding our charity from him.[28]

That the reliance on this sort of appeal alone was ill conceived can be seen from the small number of subscribers the charity attracted (only 165 by 1749), the absence of subscribers who could bring administrative talent and experience as well as financial backing to the charity, and the limited amount of financial support it received in its early years.[29]

These early subscribers to the Lock were largely of three sorts. First, there were the benevolent aristocrats and gentry, who often donated to public charities.[30] Second, in addition to support from the upper classes, the charity also received aid, either in the form of subscriptions or services, from nineteen doctors and apothecaries, who had obvious scientific and professional interests in the treatment of venereal disease. Third, there were also a significant number of military men, whose presence supports the view that the military implications of venereal disease were of growing concern during the successive wars of the mid-eighteenth century.

While the Lock Hospital hobbled through its first several decades, the Lying-in Charity continued to expand through most of the century. For example in the 1760s the charity increased the number of deliveries it assisted twelvefold – from a yearly average of only 100 in the years 1757 to 1760, to a yearly average of 1,200 between 1760 and 1769. The Lying-in Charity's efficiency undoubtedly explains its growing popularity. In the three years from 1767 to 1770 the subscription lists doubled, as the charity managed not only to attract many new donors, but also to retain most of its earlier subscribers as active, annual supporters.[31] At the Lock, however, as we have already noted, by the mid-1760s the administration of the institution had just barely survived several major crises of funding and confidence. More were to come in the next twenty years. Although income and numbers cared for increased through the mid-1780s, the end of the American War created a crisis at the Lock. Commenting on the more than 530 patients treated in the hospital in 1783 and 1784, the governors noted of 'the numerous Objects received into the Hospital', 'that many of them arrived from abroad after the close of the last War'. Preceding this massive increase in numbers cared for and pressure on hospital resources, a bitter and almost fatal conflict arose between the governors and the hospital's doctor, William Bromfield. Each blamed the other for the hospital's misfortunes. This breach was healed only partially after Bromfield's campaign on the hospital's behalf in the mid-1780s. By that time the charity was once again in the throes of severe monetary problems. A malignant fever in the wards brought the need to clean and refurnish the entire institution, while there was a decline in chapel income because of the refusal of the minister to give regular sermons. This led to 'a considerable deficiency in its Income' which by 1798 had become so serious that the hospital, 'now nearly fourteen Hundred Pounds in Debt', could care for only about half the number of patients that it had served ten years before.[32]

By the century's end, the fortunes of the two charities had levelled off. From the 1770s many writers realized that population was increasing, or concluded its size was not as significant a factor as had formerly been thought. These attacks on theories of declining population led to the reformulation of attitudes about the value of encouraging any increase in numbers. From worrying about population decline, and how population might best be supported and encouraged, population growth was first seen as a symptom, rather than an important cause, of a prosperous economy and finally as itself the prime cause of poverty.[33] Since population was seen as responding to, rather than responsible for, external economic circumstances like the amount of food available or the current demand for labour, reproduction could be left to the operations of the market.

> In this manner the demand for men, like that for any other commodity, necessarily regulates the production of men; quickens it when it goes too slowly, and stops it when it advances too fast. It is this demand which regulates and determines the state of propagation in all the different countries of the world.[34]

In addition to the effects of changes in demographic theory on support to lying-in charities there were the consequences of the loss of the American colonies. This change in Britain's imperial position, and the withdrawal of the colonies as places that demanded both settlers and defenders, decreased the felt need for a growing population of potential soldiers, sailors and colonizers. When a large population of labouring poor were seen as having little economic value, the existence of such a population assumed a triply sinister aspect. Since the poor had less productive value, since they consumed more than they produced, and since, by their improvidence and immorality, they often had bad effects on the manners and morals of society, there was no apparent reason to wish for their increase. Thus with the overthrowing of mercantilist views of the beneficial economic effects of population growth came a disdain and fear of 'mere' procreation, and of charities which encouraged this.[35]

By the 1780s the number of deliveries performed by the Lying-in Charity fell, and remained well below the level of the 1770s, increasing again only towards the end of the 1780s. In the 1790s the amount of aid given rose, but the charity started its long decline at the height of the hungry years of the 1790s. Although the number of deliveries performed by the Lying-in Charity seems to rise and fall with the London birth-rate through the late 1770s and 1780s, by 1803 the number of women it delivered had already started to plummet. This decrease in service was not a simple response to a fall in revenues, for the charity aided a very large number of women (5,035) in 1791 when available funds were quite low, and when it meant putting the charity almost £100 in the red. The reduction of women delivered in 1803 occurred despite a large increase in the charity's revenues.[36] By contrast, with the takeover of the Lock's direction by members of the Clapham Sect, that charity finally stabilized, attracting more experienced and generous subscribers. By 1798, although the Lock still listed only 147 donors, more than one-third of these gave to at least one other charity and almost a quarter to four charities or more. Four members of the Drummond family, bankers and philanthropists, were donors as well as a host of MPs and members of London's business and mercantile community. One reason for the charity's belated success was the new interest in and concern with sexual vice and disease that seemed to weigh heavily on the public mind during the French wars.[37]

The wars, often described as a spiritual counterpart of venereal infection, made both the containment of these physical diseases and the quarantine of so-called 'moral illness' of first importance. While gainful employment for women was thought to be on the wane, and as a consequence prostitution and attendant disease more common, contemporaries believed it was vital, not only for the physical well-being of the nation but also for its spiritual and moral health, that this plague be controlled. Curing people of venereal disease was not enough; the work of moral reformation was at least as important. And when in 1787 the Lock Hospital set up a sister institution, the Lock Asylum, to accomplish this reformation, the fortunes of the charity looked up. By 1803 not only had the charity attracted the attention and support of the right kinds of donors, but also its finances were stronger than they had been for thirty years.[38]

Thus we see, in the changing circumstances of both these medical charities, what uneasy allies philanthropy and medicine were. The purely medical and scientific aspects of both charities were only supported and allowed scope when they were seen to coincide with, and support, widely held views on local and national policy. Those organizations that could appeal to the prudence and good value of their enterprise, as well as to its humanity, were undoubtedly the most successful. Those charities, like the Lock, which relied primarily on appeals to disinterested benevolence, needed changes in external circumstances, like the French wars, to focus attention on their work and convince possible subscribers of the value of donation. For the largest and most important group of givers were hard-headed London businessmen who needed to be convinced of the certainty and magnitude of the returns on their invested benevolence. Whether serving as a bolster to Britain's international ambitions or as an agent of her moral rehabilitation, successful eighteenth-century London charity had always to justify itself by noting its contributions to these grander national projects.

NOTES

1 See M. G. Jones, *Hannah More*, Cambridge, 1952, and J. P. Malcolm, *Anecdotes of the Manners and Customs of London during the Eighteenth Century* [1800], 2 vols, 2nd edn, London, 1810, vol. 1, p. 16. A correspondent to the *Gentleman's Magazine*, 1747, pp. 163–4, held that 'since the Reformation has banished ignorance and restored Christianity we have nobly distinguished ourselves by donations of another kind [from those of Catholics], such as are truly stiled *charities*'.

2 This is not, however, to disparage the funds raised by bequest. See for example the records of the General Lying-in Hospital, Weekly Minute Book (1769–77), 5 July 1774. The amount of legacies and their significance in the total finances of each charity varied enormously. Furthermore, several charities lumped legacies with benefactions in their

annual reports, or made peculiar reckonings. Thus the Magdalen, in its 1776 report, noted the legacies of two subscribers who were not yet dead. What I have done is to average the known legacies of the charities in this period in terms of their percentage significance, and come up with a 20 per cent mean. Most of the remaining 80 per cent came from subscriptions.

3 B. Mandeville, *The Fable of the Bees* [1723], ed. P. Harth, Harmondsworth, 1970, pp. 269, 287, 264. Referring to mercantile sponsorships of charity schools, he wrote, 'They have no Thought of Interest, even those who deal in and provide those Children with what they want, have not the least design of getting by what they sell for their Use, and tho' in every thing else their Avarice and Greediness after Lucre be glaringly conspicuous, in this affair they are wholly divested from selfishness and have no Worldly Ends'. Mandeville was of course being vastly ironic.

4 All the Lock records are held by the Royal College of Surgeons, Lincolns Inn Fields, London.

5 W. Petty, cited in K. R. Kuczynsky, 'British demographers' opinions on fertility, 1660–1760', in L. Hogben, *Political Arithmetic*, London, 1938, p. 318; J. Addison, *The Guardian* [1713], 2 vols, London, 1714, vol. 2, pp. 125–6.

6 J. Hanway, *The Defects of Police the Cause of Immorality* . . ., London, 1775, pp. xx–xxi.

7 In the 1750s for example the British Lying-in Hospital had between twelve and fifteen medical practitioners, the City of London had between six and eight, and the Middlesex about ten.

8 Thus T. Church, *A Sermon Preached . . . Before the President and Governors of the City of London Lying Hospital for Married Women*, London, 1753, p. 20, commended the hospital for 'the utter exclusion of all pupils of surgery whose presence might shock the modesty of some and give offense to others'.

9 J. S. Lewis, 'Maternal health in the English aristocracy: myths and realities, 1790–1840', *Journal of Social History*, 1983–4, vol. 17, p. 108, notes that few babies were delivered by forceps in eighteenth-century maternity hospitals.

10 J. Leake, *A Course of Lectures on the Theory and Practice of Midwifery*, London, 1775, and Leake, *A Syllabus of Lectures on the Theory and Practice of Midwifery*, London, 1776; P. Rhodes, *Dr Leake's Hospital*, London, 1978.

11 See J. Dwyer, *Virtuous Discourse*, Edinburgh, 1987; R. S. Crane, 'Suggestions towards a genealogy of the "Man of Feelings"', *ELH*, 1934, vol. 1; Church, op. cit., p. 9.

12 J. Lawson, *Occasional Sermons*, Dublin, 1765, pp. 299–300.

13 C. Woodward, 'Reality and social reform – the transition from laissez-faire to the welfare state', *Yale Law Journal*, 1962, p. 302.

14 Church, op. cit., pp. 18–19.

15 *Gentleman's Magazine* (1769), pp. 601–2. See also Lawson, op. cit., pp. 294–6.

16 L. Braddon, *The Form of a Petition for Relieving, Reforming and Employing the Poor*, London, 1722, p. 19.

17 L. Braddon, *Particular Answers to the Most Material Objections made to the Proposal Humbly Presented to His Majesty, for Relieving, Reforming and Employing all the Poor of Great Britain*, London, 1722, pp. 10–12.

18 W. Bell, *A Dissertation on the Following Subject: What Causes principally contribute to render a nation populous? And what effect has the populousness of a nation on its Trade?*, Cambridge, 1756, pp. 33, 35. See also Bell, *Britannia Languens, or a Discourse on Trade* (1680), in J. R. McCulloch (ed.) *Early English Tracts on Commerce*, Cambridge, 1954, pp. 345–50.

19 See for example J. Aiken, *Thoughts on Hospitals*, London, 1771, p. 62.

20 *A Plain Account of the Advantages of the Lying-In Charity*, London, 1767, p. 7.

21 Ibid., p. 8.

22 B. North, *Sermon for the ... Lying-In Charity*, London, 1771, pp. 17–18, 14–15; *A Plain Account*, 1767, p. 8.

23 This may have something to do with the different class compositions of each subscriber group. Out of 303 subscribers to the British Lying-in Hospital, 54 were aristocrats, while in the Lying-in Charity there were only 10 out of 381 subscribers.

24 The words in quotations were used to describe Job Orton, whose writings were frequently distributed gratis by the Society for Promoting Christian Knowledge among the Poor. At least forty-one of the subscribers listed in the 1767 rolls of the Charity also subscribed to the SPCK.

25 Although it helped a charity to have a member of the royal family or a prince of the Church as one of its subscribers, in the long run a charity's health and good governance depended on the involvement of men of wide-ranging acquaintance and influence. Women did not sit on the governing boards of these charities until the nineteenth century.

26 See *An Account of the Proceedings of the Governors of the Lock Hospital for July 14 1746 to September 29 1749*, n. pl., 1749, for an appeal to the public against the practice of seeking out child prostitutes under the mistaken impression that intercourse with an unpolluted victim, by transmitting the disease, would cure it in the purchaser.

27 Lock Hospital General Court Book Number 1, 4 July 1746 to 29 May 1762. Meetings to be held in July and October 1756 were cancelled as were those in January, April, May and July 1757, January and March 1758, March, November and December 1759, March 1760 and again at the decade's end in August and October 1769 and January 1770.

28 M. Madan, *Sermon for the Opening of the Chapel at the Lock Hospital*, London, 1762, p. 21.

29 Within the first years of its foundation, the Lock had to dismiss two larcenous preachers. During its first five years of service, its annual income was little more than £700. Of the sixty-two men who are listed as attending directors' committee meetings before 1751, only two (John Beard to six, Nathaniel Curzon to two) have been identified as donors to more than one other charity. Three others subscribed to one other charity. An additional twelve may have either given money themselves or had a close relative subscribe: for these the information is too scanty

to be more certain.

30 Martin Madan, one of the founders of the Lock, may have contributed to the support of this charity received from the upper classes. His own antecedents and connections were highly respectable. His father was an MP, his grandfather a judge, and his younger brother, Spencer Madan, became bishop of Peterborough.

31 *A Plain Account*, 1767. The Lying-in's 1770 subscription list contained only 29 aristocratic names (about 4 per cent of 603 subscribers).

32 The Select Committee of the Lock, in order to fight Bromfield's influence, put advertisements in the newspapers advising subscribers and supporters of the hospital to disregard the cards sent around by Bromfield, and to continue their contributions to 'this most useful and humane Charity': *The Times*, 18 March 1782, p. 1. The Lock Hospital General Court Book Number 3 (April 1773 to March 1789), esp. pp. 108–14; and Number 4 (April 1789 to March 1816), p. 88.

33 J. Townsend, *A Dissertation on the Poor Laws*, 1797 (reprint Berkeley, Calif., 1971), p. 46. 'The farmer breeds only from the best of all his cattle; but our laws choose rather to preserve the worst, and seem anxious lest the breed should fail.' J. Howlett, *Examination of Mr Pitt's Speech . . . Relative to the Condition of the Poor*, London, 1796, pp. 28–9. Howlett (1731–1804) was best known as a statistician and political economist.

34 A. Smith, *The Wealth of Nations* (1776), ed. E. Cannan, 2 vols, London, 1961, vol. 1, p. 62. See also J. Steuart, *An Inquiry into the Principles of Political Economy* (1767), ed. A. S. Skinner, 2 vols, Chicago, 1966, vol. 1, p. 32.

35 T. Mortimer, *Lectures on the Elements of Commerce, Politics and Finance* (1772), London, 1801, p. 105. In *Political Observations on the Population of Countries*, London, 1782, p. 3, it is noted that a large population is not even needed for national power and self defence.

36 The Lying-in Charity delivered a record number of 5,035 women in one year in 1791 despite the fact that its expenditure amounted to £1,559 and its income to only £1,500. In 1803, when it delivered 4,473 women, it had invested £537 in stocks and had a balance of more than £300 in hand. See *An Account of the Lying-in Charity*, 1791, 1803.

37 For fuller details, see R. Soloway, 'Reform or ruin: English moral thought during the first French Republic', *The Review of Politics*, 1963, and chapter 6 of D. Andrew, *Philanthropy and Police: London Charity in the Eighteenth Century*, Princeton, NJ, 1989.

38 See the Lock Hospital's General Court Book Number 4 (April 1789 to March 1816).

6

THE *SOCIETE DE CHARITE MATERNELLE*, 1788–1815

Stuart Woolf

Childbirth and infancy have been privileged subjects of charity at least since the foundling hospitals of the later Middle Ages. In the later eighteenth century the pregnant mother and the newborn enjoyed pride of place among the categories of the poor whose condition aroused compassion, concern and even assistance. For the philosophers, such as Diderot, the role of women was marriage and reproduction. For painters like Greuze and Chardin, who popularized a new artistic genre, the good and beloved mother was the linchpin of the happy family, which reflected the order of nature. Childbirth bridged the private and public spheres. For while the act of parturition remained cloaked in ritual and symbolism, human reproduction extended far beyond the household, investing the language and practices of society and the intervention of the state. Morals, law, power and authority were inextricably involved in the debates on child abandonment and infanticide, population and national strength, midwifery and the female anatomy: their chosen arena was childbirth. Medical discussions and experiments to improve the survival chances of mother and newborn – through breast-feeding or vaccination – could be considered as affecting all society and hence as bridging the social divide. But in general both language and practice were concerned with the bodies of the poor, in literature and painting as much as in the caesarian section experimented with in France or the wax anatomical specimens modelled at Florence in the 1780s.[1]

The counterpart to the morbid interest in the female body and sexuality so characteristic of the later eighteenth century was the representation of the poor mother and child as innocent victims of a corrupt society. The abandoned mother, topos of the literature of these decades, was matched by the 'fancy pictures' of poor children of Reynolds and Gainsborough. The mother was paradigmatic of the virtues of an idealized image of the laborious poor, contrasted in their frugality, simplicity and physical health (at least in rural settings) to the luxury, corruption and ailments of the idle rich. The religious symbolism of the innocence of infants and the humanity that had always imbued charitable action reinforced the more recent pedagogic beliefs inspired by Locke and Rousseau in the possibilities of imprinting and shaping the newborn child. Mother and children, in large families, were recounted in French morality stories in the 1780s as exemplary objects of *bienfaisance*. Medical practitioners like Tissot attributed the poor health of infants to the excessive workload of mothers while pregnant. And behind this social concern for the particular vulnerability of the protagonists of childbirth, the age-old utilitarian argument about the importance to the state of the survival of infants (including bastards) was regularly voiced.[2]

The immediate context of the Parisian Society for Maternal Charity was provided by the debates about abandoned infants and breast-feeding. The issue of foundling hospitals and in particular the question of the so-called *tours* (which allowed mothers to retain anonymity when abandoning their children) had become a lively one throughout western Europe by the later eighteenth century. The increase in abandonment was related not to demographic growth, but to the ease of access to foundling hospitals, and the extremely high level of infant mortality was blamed on hospital conditions. The critique of foundling hospitals formed part of a more general rationalistic Enlightenment attack on charity and charitable institutions, regarded as generating the poor by their very existence; while the evidence of infant mortality was deployed as a weapon in a broader campaign against hospitalization in contrast to outdoor assistance at home. The Paris Hôpital Général contained the largest foundling hospital in Europe, attracting between 5,500 and 7,500 abandoned infants a year by *c.*1780 from all over northern France; all contemporaries agreed that at least two-thirds died in their first year, and far more by the age of 7.[3] Precisely because of the enormous pressures and difficulties in feeding the foundlings, medical practitioners had experimented in the 1780s with alternative methods of artificial nutrition. Among the philanthropists funding such efforts in the early 1780s was Mme Fougeret, the founder of the Society for Maternal Charity. The results of all these experiments had proved disastrous, with almost total mortality, so reinforcing the arguments in favour of breast-feeding.[4]

The Society for Maternal Charity was a typical creation of the end of the old regime in France, in which humanity was closely allied to that practical religiosity which identified itself in the tradition of St Vincent de Paul. It resembled other voluntary associations founded in the 1780s, like the Philanthropic Society of Paris or similar societies in major provincial cities, especially Lyon.[5] Its early history is unusually well documented, because it was caught up in the whirlpool of the Revolution and subsequent Napoleonic normalization. The society is of considerable interest to the study of the relationship between charity and medicine, not only because it offers the opportunity to compare representations of medical charity to their practice, but also through the insights it provides into the role of women, the relationship between public and private assistance, and the forms of mediation intrinsic to the activities of all private charities. Despite the major political ruptures of French history, the survival of the society until the late 1870s (when its activities were presumably absorbed within state welfare provision) points to continuity in mentalities from the old regime through to the Restoration.[6]

The society was founded in May 1788. Its purpose – as its officers explained to the Committee of Mendicity of the Constituent Assembly in July 1790 – was to assist 'a class of poor for whom there are neither hospitals nor foundations at Paris – namely, the legitimate infants of the poor'. The primary reason for such assistance was to prevent parents from either abandoning their newborn, or using the municipal lying-in facilities, whether at the Hôtel-Dieu (which could easily prove fatal for mother and infant) or at the Wet-nurse Bureau (whose charges led to indebtedness and prison). There were, according to the ladies of the society, at least 800 legitimate infants left annually at the Foundling Hospital (a figure calculated as 1,200–1,400 by 1804), where overcrowding, disease and shortage of resources led to high mortality, estimated at two-thirds of all infants.

The Society for Maternal Charity aimed at persuading married working mothers to give birth and to breast-feed at home by the provision of financial and personal assistance. It is worth quoting at length the moral arguments proposed by the president, the duchess Cossé, in her presentation of the society to Marie Antoinette at Versailles on 4 January 1790:[7]

to recall to nature hapless mothers, degraded by poverty, who abandon their infants as if they were the sad fruits of disorder; to bring to an end this inhuman abuse; to give back to morality [*moeurs*] a multitude of families and to the state a numerous population lost in the hospitals. . . . [This means] an important revolution in the habits [*moeurs*] of the people, to be achieved through persuasion, example and the tender consolations of charity. . . . One should pity rather than reject a people degraded by its vices and excesses, which are the fruits of despair and wretchedness. Superior and enlightened reason is needed to demonstrate that the people, too often devoid of principles, can only be recalled to virtue by practising the duties of nature. Nature will have won when men no longer break their sacred bonds without remorse, when it will have made men virtuous, who will no longer dishonour their titles of husband and father.

The language of the discourse is revealing, with its opposition of 'nature' to 'disorder', 'hapless mothers' to 'dishonourable husbands', the ambivalence of the term '*moeurs*' as the definition both of superior morality and of the unprincipled habits of the people, the presumption that the family was the natural core of society, but the implication that it was easily subject to conflict. There was a candid recognition of the relationship between poverty and size of family, stated most explicitly in a later report: 'infants died in families whose fecundity worsened their indigence'.[8] The people, but especially mothers, ignorant but fundamentally innocent, whose undesirable practices were attributable to their wretched material conditions, could be restored to the order of nature, in the shape of the family, by charitable action.

The discourse formed part of the new image attributed to women in the later eighteenth century, a femininity at one with nature in its attributes of modesty, tender feelings and morality. Within the broad, complex and ambiguous debate about the specificity of womanhood, carried on overwhelmingly by male exponents of the Enlightenment, maternal charity was universally recognized as appertaining to the sphere of women. Duchess Cossé's speech to the Queen might be regarded as a mere rhetorical figure of speech, given that Marie Antoinette was reputed to have expressed her desire 'to live as a mother, to feed my child and devote myself to its upbringing'.[9] Indeed, only six months later, in their appeal for support to the male Committee of Mendicity of the Constituent Assembly, the same ladies spoke of 'this violation of the sacred rights of *paternity* [my emphasis] committed daily by the poor of Paris, which appears as a disorder that needs to be fought against, out of respect for morality [*moeurs*]'.[10] But from the outset, the founding members were clear that they constituted an association of women. Indeed they offer an explanation which, in its very contradiction to the later-eighteenth-century idealization of the fragility and delicacy of the weaker sex, expresses the ambivalence of the debate on the nature of womanhood. They claimed as specific to the female sex, particularly in relation to the bond between mother and child, the quality of sensibility, a term charged with physiological and social significance by writers like Cabanis:[11] 'Providence has called women in particular to the help of infants and indigent mothers, because their sensibility makes it easier for them to overcome the disgust surrounding the squalor of poverty'.[12]

In fact initially, alongside 145 ladies, there were 48 male subscribing members, as well as 63 others who made donations. In 1809 there were 134 women and 40 men. But apart from the treasurer (necessarily a man), the organization, administration and running of the society were and remained exclusively in the hands of women. Victim of the Jacobin suppression of all associations in 1793, the society not only remained a female domain on its resuscitation in 1800, but also became the official embodiment of the natural affinity for charitable work attributed to women, when Napoleon transformed it into an exclusive Court club under the presidency of the empress Marie Louise (1810). The Society for Maternal Charity provides an early example of that characteristic occupation by upper- and middle-class ladies of the only public space – charitable activities – permitted them in the nineteenth century.

But, like their successors, the ladies of our society could operate in a male world only through their network of relatives. The membership of the society in its earliest years provides an excellent indicator of the conduits of its financial success in the shadow of the Court and Constituent Assembly. Its founder, Mme Fougeret, was the daughter of a lawyer, wife of a *receveur général des finances* and mother-in-law of a president of the *Cour des aides*, who acted as treasurer. Its members included the wives of leading Court administrative and scientific figures of the pre-Revolutionary and Revolutionary years: nobles such as the duchesses Cossé and

France de Croisset, marquise de Montagne, comtesse Le Camus, alongside the wives of the ministers Necker, D'Ormesson and the tax-farmer and scientist Lavoisier. The most assiduous attenders at the weekly meetings (held in the Foundling Hospital) were the wives of mostly unknown but wealthy men, with a bias towards *fonctionnaires* (Pastoret, Marcilly, Vergennes, Vernon, Frileuse, Dupont de Nemours, Grivel, and others). It was Necker who presented the society to Marie Antoinette, who then assigned it an annual income of 24,000 livres (about a quarter of its expenditure). It was certainly through these Court connections that the Philanthropic Society, under Béthune-Charost, agreed to subsidize a new category, of artisan families with at least five children, at an annual cost of 1,200 livres. It was the same inner network of connections that helps explain the decisive support of the president of the Committee of Mendicity, La Rochefoucauld-Liancourt, that ensured the society – unique among such associations, where even the Philanthropic Society was refused – an income voted by the National Assembly. Nor is it surprising that this voluntary society, rather than some other, should have been so honoured by Napoleon, when one considers that its administrative committee in 1810 included the wives of imperial ministers, senators and administrators like Champagny, Chaptal, Cretet, Choiseul, Delessert, Gérando, Béthune-Charost and Montmorency.[13]

Realistic in their sense of the practical limits to their capacity to do good, the worthy ladies displayed a notable modernity in their identification of family needs. Two groups were recognized as particularly vulnerable. The first consisted of families whose household income was at risk: pregnant women, with at least one surviving child, whose husband had died or fallen ill; or women with at least two living children, who had themselves fallen ill. The second comprised large families, with at least three surviving children aged under 14; particularly noteworthy is the recognition that the children in such large families would often be the offspring of successive marriages. The subsidy from the Philanthropic Society reinforced this analysis of family needs, as it was limited to pregnant widows with at least five living children and also included professional training for boys till the age of 14. The condition of abandoned women was appropriately regarded as equivalent to that of the widow: 'these unhappy victims of the disorder of their husbands, who find themselves alone, after all their possessions have been dissipated, without a bed, without clothing, surrounded by infants sleeping on straw, about to give birth to another hapless babe'.[14]

The means by which the society intervened were economic and moral. Public health and preventive issues were certainly implicit, although in a strict sense the society's mode of action only marginally involved direct medical intervention. No medical practitioners were involved, nor is there ever any mention of midwives. In the Napoleonic Society, each mother was allowed a small credit of 10 francs for medicines and obliged to vaccinate her infant.[15] Otherwise life and death were presented as black and white alternatives, with barely any recognition of illness. Only if a mother's sickness prevented her from breast-feeding was a doctor or a surgeon called in, not to cure but to check the need for a wet-nurse. The very mention of a surgeon, a lower category of medical practitioner, was indicative of the marginal role attributed by the society to the medical profession or at least its refusal to contemplate expenditure for medical care. The mother received 18 livres to cover her accouchement and a layette, costed at 20 livres. She was then paid a monthly subsidy of 8 livres for the first year and 4 livres for the second year, on condition that she breast-fed her child (or had the child breast-fed if she were unable to). These twenty-four months corresponded to the expected period of lactation, but the ladies of the society hoped to subsidize the mothers for a third year. No more details are given, leaving the historian with tantalizing questions. Was the extension to a third year – which implied an unusually lengthy period of breast-feeding – seen as a means to delay fertility? What work patterns were envisaged that would have corresponded to the gradually diminishing level of subsidy?

Great stress was placed on the relationship between donor and recipient, structured around visits to the mother's home. Such personal contact and control was not unusual: the London Foundling Hospital officials, for example, called on the homes where their children were cared for. Indeed personal visitations were soon to be theorized by Gérando and adopted as the standard mould of nineteenth-century voluntary charity.[16] It was the duty of the ladies, in the district of Paris for which each was responsible, to visit the mothers who requested help and check on their credentials before presenting the case to the committee. As always in charitable operations, a superficially transparent system masked an opaque layer of social relations. Among the ladies themselves, a distinction was made between the 'deputies' of the committee and the *dames administrantes*, only the latter carrying out visitations. Not surprisingly the lady deputies tended to be of higher social rank: it was Mme Lavoisier, not the duchess de Crosne, who lifted her skirts to step over the effluent of the faubourg St Antoine.

Less clear is how the mothers were chosen. The society insisted on certain criteria that effectively delimited the pool of potential applicants: they had to be married women, of good repute, domiciled in Paris for at least one year. The qualifications of respectability and local residence were essential features of the conventional identikit of the deserving. The ladies of the society shared that obsessive fear (characteristic of modern charity) of deceit which personal visits were meant to detect. Mme Lavoisier, for example,

> said that she had a denunciation to make, she had found out that the woman Dorleans, whom she had admitted on 24 July 1789 as number 419, had made a false declaration that she had six children. The committee decided that the woman Dorleans should forfeit the help of the Society instantly and for the future.[17]

But the very qualifications excluded the overwhelming majority of women who came to the Foundling Hospital for their accouchement or abandoned their newborn infant, as they were unmarried or came to Paris from its vast hinterland.

It was universally acknowledged that choice had to be made, given the ubiquity of poverty. Medical opinion was hardly ever sought, as it was not health, but merit, economic need and utility that provided the guidelines. Indeed ill-health was probably considered a handicap, as it increased dangers of parturition and might lead to infection. Thus sick pregnant women had to provide a certificate from a medical practitioner, while the layette was left with the mother of a dead infant explicitly because of dangers of infection. Utility and economic needs were so important that the society refused to allow the allocation of subsidies in the wealthier districts of Paris to be used for women in the poorer districts who did not exactly meet their specifications, as this would merely raise expectations and hence requests for help.[18] How the mothers heard about the society remains obscure. One can only surmise that information was passed on by parish priest, street spokesman or neighbour or spread by word of mouth. This would have been all the easier, given the localized responsibilities of the society's ladies. In this respect the society conformed to the working practices of presumably most outdoor charitable initiatives, as assistance 'at home' implied a street-to-street basis. The demand was evidently high, for duchess Cossé told Marie Antoinette that over 1,500 mothers had been rejected in the first eight months. The women were required to present their marriage certificate and a written declaration of good conduct, whereas an oral declaration was enough to confirm their Parisian domicile. Standard referees were listed for the character testimonial – the parish priest, neighbours, the main landlord of the building. What we are offered by these snippets of information is a glimpse into an essentially unknown and perhaps unknowable world of social relations in crowded living quarters, where a premium was placed on respectable, pacific and amicable comportment and a high degree of dependence on neighbours.

The register of women assisted in the 1780s allows us to identify the social physiognomy of the families, as well as their topographical distribution, for it includes details of the numbers of children in each family and the husband's profession. As the ladies of the society recognized, the most populous districts of Paris – St Antoine and St Marceau – were those of greatest need, and to these were allocated a larger number of grants and a second fieldworker to carry out the visits. There were families with as few as two and as many as ten children, but the great majority had between three and five: a random sample of 224 families (19 per cent of the total number in the register) shows an average 4.3 children per family. The trades were typically those of the Parisian labouring classes: cobblers, coachmen, bricklayers, *gagne-deniers*, water-carriers, carpenters, stone-cutters, fruit-sellers, gardeners and cow-keepers, ebony- and bone-carvers, carders and fan-makers, wig-makers and hatters, scribes and measurers, and the infinite number of other ways of making a living, with the occasional decayed master and more numerous journeymen and apprentices. The social world to which the ladies of the society turned was that of the *sans-culottes*, that multitude of small artisans and petty retailers, suppliers of services, as well as casual labourers.[19] It was their very number that explained the need for testimonials and personal visits. For only so was it possible to identify the deserving amidst such an anonymous, unknown (and hence potentially deceitful) mass.

The number of women assisted depended on the funds available. In the first eighteen months (1788–9), 760 mothers were helped, an average of 42 a month; between 1790 and 1792, with the sharp reduction of funds caused by the Revolutionary upheavals, the numbers fell to between 24 and 30 a month, rising in the final three months of the society's existence in 1793 (certainly reading the writing on the wall) to 59 a month. In this first period of nearly five years a total of 1,902 mothers (an average of just over 33 per month) were assisted. With its revival in 1800, the society stayed initially at the level of about 300 annually, rising to 500 from 1804 to 1806, 450 in 1807, 300 in both 1808 and 1809 and 350 in 1810. Over these ten years, an average of 403 women were helped annually. With its elevation into the Empress's Society, the level was raised to 500 a year. The population of Paris, over 700,000 at the outbreak of the Revolution, falling to 550,000 by 1796, grew by 160,000 during the Napoleonic years.

The numbers were relatively small, compared to the society's estimates of married women going to the Foundling Hospital, and even smaller compared to the apparent demand. But the major justification of the society's activities was the sharp fall in mortality rates. In the early years (1788–93), according to the society, of the babies for which it assumed responsibility only one-fifth died, compared to two-thirds in the Foundling Hospital. In the decade 1801–10, the death-rate was 22 per cent, even though expenditure had been reduced, with typical Napoleonic economizing. The fall in costs had been achieved primarily by an abandonment of the ideal of a prolonged period of breast-feeding, with a restriction of subsidies to periods of only fifteen months. Even so, the ladies of the society could claim to have achieved their aim of reducing infant mortality (as well as that of the mothers, for whom virtually no deaths were reported) through breast-feeding.

The Society for Maternal Charity offers an example of the function of voluntary charities even in a society and period when the state claimed for itself a central and highly active role. In the earliest, most generous and utopian phase of the Revolution, the Committee of Mendicity had reached the conclusion that poor families had the right to assistance. But this did not imply the exclusion of private charity, merely a refusal of public subsidies to voluntary organizations. As La Rochefoucauld-Liancourt explained, in rejecting the appeal of the Philanthropic Society for the continuation of its former royal subsidy:

Unquestionably philanthropic societies must be encouraged and supported, for they spread individual charity with rare care, intelligence and virtue. . . . Even more, they economise infinitely on public assistance and animate private charity without which public charity would be incomplete.[20]

The fact that the Society for Maternal Charity still received a subsidy (justified on formalistic and specious legal grounds) is strong circumstantial evidence of the uniquely moral quality attributed to infant life. One can add that it served a further function – similar to that of doctors in the nineteenth century – as a source of intimate local knowledge of the labouring classes with an appropriate street-level organizational structure that could be utilized in times of emergency. It was not fortuitous that Marie Antoinette entrusted the society with a substantial sum in December 1790 to provide food, clothing, blankets, fuel and even cash to needy Parisian families during the winter of 1790–91.[21]

The complementary role of the charity, relative to the centrality of the public hospital, never changed. In the early Consulate years, the society fitted easily into the philanthropic humanitarianism that was a characteristic of Chaptal's years as Minister of the Interior.[22] But when it was taken over by Napoleon in 1810, the administration was quite clear that the society must remain complementary to the public hospitals. After elaborate calculations about the probable total number of legitimate infants at risk in Paris – estimated at 2,600 annually – Montalivet, Minister of the Interior, concluded that the survival rate of abandoned infants was much higher than before the Revolution, and that parents were no longer imprisoned for debts owed to the Bureau of Wet-nurses. But broader social reasons explain his advice against extending the role of the Society for Maternal Charity at the expense of the two public institutions, by providing it with resources to ensure home breast-feeding for all:

It is embarrassing to have to admit that there are parents who are so brutalised by vice and poverty that their infants are far more abandoned in their hands than in public institutions. This seems to have been recognised by the ladies who founded the Society, in their insistence as first condition of acceptance for aid that the fathers and mothers provide a good home.

The encouragement this Society gives to maternal virtues will undoubtedly help considerably in reforming the domestic practices [*moeurs*] of the class they assist. But it would be a dangerous illusion to believe that such a reform could happen instantly and completely. Until such a time, institutions which allow for the placement of a certain number of infants outside the paternal home merit special protection as they, more than any others, protect these infants. One also needs to bear in mind that a large number of women of the popular class cannot feed their infants as their work, like that of their husbands, is necessary for their subsistence and this work requires travel which is incompatible with the needs of breast-feeding. For such women it is clear that nothing can replace the resources that they find in the Wetnurse Bureau.[23]

It is questionable whether the society, once taken over by the Napoleonic Court, can be properly considered as a voluntary charity. It became an appendage of the imperial administration, with three princesses, seventy-three wives of grand officers, ministers, senators and councillors of state (from duchesses down), forty wives of civil and military functionaries and fifty-six other Parisian ladies. It was proposed to extend it to all the departments. The prefects displayed their zeal by recruiting their own wives and those of their closest collaborators. But they were successful in only fifty-three departments, primarily because in the others there were no large, wealthy towns, the precondition for philanthropy. By the end of the empire, membership of the society read like a roll-call of its most aristocratic, rich and socially prominent notables, whose names and qualities had been carefully vented at Paris. Perhaps the strongest link with the charitable tradition was the insistence on the discretionary character of its assistance, not to allow the poor 'to envisage as a right what is only a favour, and as an obligation what is dependent on choice by the ladies'.[24]

With the Restoration and the explicitly ideological withdrawal of the state, once more the Society for Maternal Charity survived, in its multiple civic replications, albeit on a primarily voluntary basis: 'His Majesty believes that the more respectable the purpose of the Maternal Societies, the less the Administration should use its authority to form them. Charity should not be commanded.' Even so, the sacral nature of infant life still merited small official subsidies.[25] But by now the concerns of Restoration philanthropy had spread wider. It was no accident that two of the founder members of the Society for Maternal Charity, Mme Fougeret and Mme Pastoret, should have established nurseries in their own homes for the education of poor children.[26] Breast-feeding was no longer enough.

Acknowledgement

I wish to thank Ludmilla Jordanova for her helpful comments on an earlier version of this chapter.

NOTES

1 L. J. Jordanova, 'Naturalizing the family: literature and the bio-medical sciences in the late eighteenth century', in Jordanova (ed.) *Languages of Nature*, London, 1986; Jordanova, 'La Donna di cera', *Kos*, 1984, vol. 1; D. G. Charlton, *New Images of the Natural in France*, Cambridge, 1984; E. Jacobs, 'Diderot and the education of girls', in E. Jacobs *et al.* (eds) *Women and Society in Eighteenth Century France*, London, 1979; C. Duncan, 'Happy mothers and other new ideas in French art', *Art Bulletin*, 1973, vol. 60; Y.-M. Bercé, *Le Chaudron et la lancette. Croyances populaires et médecine préventive (1798–1830)*, Paris, 1984; M.-F. Morel, 'A quoi servent les enfants trouvés? Les médecins et le problème de l'abandon dans la France du XVIIIe siècle', *Colloque 'Enfance Abandonnée et Société en Europe, XIVe–XXe siècles'*, Ecole Française de Rome, 30–31 January 1987; V. Fildes, *Breasts, Bottles and Babies*, Edinburgh, 1985.

2 J. Barrell, *The Dark Side of the Landscape. The Rural Poor in English Painting 1730–1940*, Cambridge, 1983; H. Chisick, *The Limits of Reform in the Enlightenment: Attitudes towards the Education of the Lower Class in Eighteenth Century France*, Princeton, NJ, 1981, pp. 231–2, 249, 254.

3 A. Forrest, *The French Revolution and the Poor*, Oxford, 1981, pp. 119–22; C. Bloch, *L'Assistance et l'Etat en France à la veille de la Révolution*, Paris, 1908, p. 110; G. Rosen, 'A slaughter of innocents: aspects of child health in the eighteenth-century city', *Studies in Eighteenth Century Culture*, 1976, vol. 5.

4 Morel, 'A quoi servent les enfants trouvés?'

5 The 'Société de Bienfaisance Maternelle' of Lyon claimed precedence, asserting that the Parisian society was created in imitation: C. Bloch and A. Tuetey (eds) *Procès-verbaux et rapports du Comité de Mendicité de la Constituante 1790–1791*, Paris, 1911, 20 August and 11 October 1790.

6 The main documentation on the Société de Charité Maternelle is to be found in Archives Nationales, Paris (hereafter AN), F¹⁵²565 and AF IV 450 and 451; Bibliothèque Historique de la Ville de Paris (hereafter BHVP), MSS 995, rés. 34, register with minutes of the meetings from 4 January 1790 to 19 February 1793 (I wish to thank Angela Groppi for bringing this register to my attention); Bibliothèque Nationale, Paris (hereafter BN), Fonds français 11368 and 11369 (minutes of meetings from 22 December 1810 to 25 May 1814, and correspondence). The minutes of the first forty-eight meetings (1788–9) may be in the papers of the Comité de Mendicité; the report of this committee and decisions of the National Assembly relating to the society are in Bloch and Tuetey, *Procès-verbaux*, pp. 94–6, 105, 191, 228, 230, 594–5, 693–703, 767. The register of the Imperial Society is in AN, F¹⁵²; correspondence with the departments is scattered through the departmental cartons of F¹⁵, as well as in departmental archives both in France and in the annexed regions: for example for the Arno (Tuscany) in Archivio di Stato di Firenze, Prefettura dell'Arno, 505; cf. for Hérault, C. Jones, *Charity and Bienfaisance: The Treatment of the Poor in the Montpellier Region*, Cambridge, 1982, pp. 237–9. The last published reports of various civic Societies for Maternal Charity (Dijon, Lyon, etc.) are for 1876–9: AN, F¹⁵³799 à 13805.

7 BHVP, MSS 995, rés. 34, 4 January 1790.

8 AN, F¹⁵²565, report of 1813.

9 J. McManners, *Death and the Enlightenment*, Oxford, 1981, p. 54; Charlton, op. cit., pp. 154–61.

10 Bloch and Tuetey, op. cit., p. 699.

11 Jordanova, 1986, op. cit., pp. 96–9.

12 AN, AF IV 450, no. 3396.

13 The membership of the pre-1793 years is in the minutes for 1790–3 and that for 1810–14 is listed in BHVP, MSS 995 (cited in note 7) as well as AN, F¹⁵²565, 18 January 1810.

14 BHVP, MSS 995, rés. 34, 4 January 1790.

15 BN, Fonds français, 11368, 23 November 1811.

16 J.-M. de Gérando, *Le Visiteur du Pauvre*, Paris, 1820, 4th edn, 1837; English translation: *The Visitor of the Poor*, London, 1833.

17 BHVP, MSS 995, rés. 34, 20 February 1790. On criteria for identification of the deserving, see S. Woolf, *The Poor in Western Europe in the Eighteenth and Nineteenth Centuries*, London, 1986.

18 BHVP, MSS 995, rés. 34, 19 February 1793.

19 For a more detailed analysis of this social level of Parisian inhabitants, see A. Groppi, *La Classe la plus nombreuse, la plus utile et la plus précieuse: Organizzazione del lavoro e conflitti nella Parigi rivoluzionaria*, EUI Working Paper no. 88/325, Florence, 1988.

20 A. Tuetey, *L'Assistance publique à Paris pendant la Révolution*, Paris, 1895, vol. 1, pp. 37–8.

21 BHVP, MSS 995, rés. 34, 13 December 1790. The sum of 66,000 livres was over twice the Queen's initial grant for the society's normal purposes. During the terrible winter of 1812, the Napoleonic administration was to use the main outdoor charity at Florence, the

Congregation of San Giovanni Battista, for exactly the same reasons, to distribute daily soup rations: Woolf, op. cit., pp. 92–3, 160.

22 It was in these years that A. Duquesnoy, *éminence grise* of the ministry, translated and published a *Recueil des mémoires sur les établissements de l'humanité* in 18 volumes (Paris, ans VII–XIII).

23 AN, AF IV 451, no. 3397.

24 BN, Fonds français, 11368, 19 March 1812.

25 AN, F15 2526, 19 December 1814.

26 BN, Fonds français, 11368, 29 November 1813; L. Passerini, *Storia degli stabilimenti di beneficenza e d'istruzione elementare gratuita della città di Firenze*, Florence, 1853, pp. 757–8.

7

URBAN GROWTH AND MEDICAL CHARITY

Hamburg 1788–1815

Mary Lindemann

There are few studies which address relationships between urban growth and charity in the eighteenth century, compared to the range of work on this theme for the nineteenth century. In the earlier period other questions have dominated, for example the impact of religious reform and humanism on charity. This deficiency is particularly striking, first because urbanization was a key factor in the redefinition of charity in the eighteenth (and perhaps also in the seventeenth) century, and second, because eighteenth-century reformers themselves were acutely aware of the implications of urban size and especially of population growth for the formulation of social policies. Germany in the eighteenth century has enjoyed far less attention from social and urban historians than either Britain or France. Perhaps this is because one does not usually think of Germany as a land of thriving cities: our vision is more bucolic and rustic. Moreover, the lack of interest probably stems as well from the mistaken beliefs that Germany in the eighteenth century was still a shattered land, barely moving on the road to recovery after the devastation of the Thirty Years' War, and that Germany until the mid-nineteenth century merely stumbled along in the wake of western European developments. Yet while Germany boasted of no metropolises to compare with London and Paris, there were numerous cities which were even then afflicted with the problems and, as we should not forget, also blessed by the advantages of urbanization. Vienna and Berlin were major cities; Frankfurt and Munich, although much smaller, were not insignificant dots on a rural landscape. But perhaps the one city in Germany, indeed in all of central Europe, whose development paralleled most closely that of London and Paris, or of Amsterdam and Antwerp, was Hamburg. Hamburg in the eighteenth century began to experience all the problems of urbanization with which urban and medical historians are so familiar: an influx of population, growing human diversity, overtaxed sanitary facilities, acute deficiencies in housing and transportation. Urbanization dictated not only a new etiquette of city life, but also new governmental practices, new and expensive municipal responsibilities, and new directions in charity.[1] Urbanization in the eighteenth century, therefore, as much as religious upheaval in the sixteenth, entailed a restructuring of charity that included medical care.

Hamburg, like most other large cities, boasted a panoply of 'spitals' either inherited from the Middle Ages or constructed in the sixteenth and seventeenth centuries.[2] These were themselves products of earlier, smaller waves of urbanization. But, despite the considerable size and often generous endowment of such institutions, they were increasingly unable to deal with the by-products of the 'new' urban growth of the eighteenth century.

Over the course of two centuries Hamburg had become a trade emporium rivalled in northern Europe only by Amsterdam and Antwerp. Until the mid-eighteenth century Hamburg had successfully mixed manufacturing for export, production for the home market, and commerce. The proportions were always uneven and commerce had always dominated; but beginning in the late seventeenth century, and even more obviously in the next hundred years, overseas commerce and the manufactories which produced for export – calico printing, sugar refining, tobacco processing – undercut the importance of the other branches of the economy. Hamburg's prosperity and the well-being of its working and trading populations became ever more dependent on the vagaries of world trade and tremulously sensitive to any wavering in its progress.

The composition of the labouring class had changed as well. Commerce, the export trades that predominated, and the booming construction industry – all characteristic of Hamburg's pattern of urbanization – relied on thousands of unskilled or semi-skilled labourers. The city's burgeoning population – over 100,000 by 1787 – in turn demanded ever more goods and services that the guilds alone could no longer supply, thereby allowing non-guilded artisans and workers a wider place in the labour-market. Thus the labouring class that existed after 1750 in Hamburg included more recent immigrants and more transients, more aliens and fewer citizens, than ever before.

Simply put, a new class of the labouring poor – the *arbeitende Arme* – had developed. The fortunes of the labouring classes came to be closely linked to something they could not control: commerce. The precariousness of labourers' lives, their perilous dance on the brink of impoverishment, did not go unrecognized by the reformers of the late eighteenth century. These men came to believe that most poverty was neither culpable nor self-induced. Rather the workings of a 'modern' economy, in particular the workings of Hamburg's economy, made it virtually impossible for labourers to avoid cycles of destitution from which they often failed to recover. Caspar Voght, one of the founding fathers of the General Poor Relief established in 1788 in Hamburg, and one of the most influential figures in poor relief reform in Europe, regarded only a minority of the poor as 'guilty' of their poverty, that is as products of 'incapacity, folly, and vice'. 'I am afraid,' he pointed out to an English audience in 1796,

> that by far the greatest number of poor in Europe is of a very different description. . . . Through a concurrence of numerous circumstances, the price of labour and of the necessaries of life is in a very unfavorable proportion for the poor in most countries of Europe.[3]

And even though these men were all (or almost all) economic liberals and free-traders, they also practised a civic paternalism that called for state intervention into some matters, most clearly social welfare policies, whenever and wherever 'disequilibriums' evidenced themselves. At the same time, they recognized that the labouring poor had become indispensable to the workings of Hamburg's economy and that helping them avoid impoverishment was an important communal obligation that the state and its citizens shirked only at great peril to their own socio-economic and moral well-being. The rise of a new sort of medical charity in Hamburg is closely connected to this perception of the new poor and of the vital role they had come to play in Hamburg's economic life.

Likewise, throughout Europe, health care and hospital reform were closely linked to poor relief reform and were driven by similar economic factors. The 'deathtraps for the poor', as hospitals were often held to be,[4] threatened plans that cherished an industrious and numerous population as the *sine qua non* of economic prosperity and as the true measure of the wealth and power of a state. Such patterns of thought ultimately endowed the people with an enhanced worth gauged directly to their actual or potential productive capacities.

The French physiocrats, the English political arithmeticians and the German cameralists, as well as most representatives of the German Enlightenment, had come to regard common labourers, rural or urban, as national assets and mainstays of the economy.[5]

The dissemination and acceptance of this point of view, combined with an increasingly grievous and more visible impoverishment, especially in the cities, stimulated much-needed redefinitions of poverty and social welfare. The definition of poverty, for instance, underwent a crucial metamorphosis and the term 'poor' came to be used routinely when speaking of a larger section of the population than merely the destitute. Poor relief reforms initiated in the closing decades of the eighteenth century directed their efforts more and more toward a new and more numerous poor, a group that equalled the labouring poor or potential poor (Jean Gutton's *paupérisable*). Nowhere was this transformation more obvious than in bustling commercial centres of which Hamburg was undeniably the premier German example. Here the problem of poverty had grown steadily throughout the 1770s and 1780s and had evoked criticism of traditional and no longer adequate forms of poor relief.[6]

The existence of a direct tie between poverty and disease, or rather between disease and impoverishment, was widely accepted. Medical and charitable reformers both spoke by no means hypocritically of 'the reduction of human suffering' as their highest goal, and of humanitarianism as their sole motivation. Yet no one lost sight of the need to 'preserve the lives of the poor [who] . . . are the hardest workers and thus most valuable to the state'.[7] Considerations of 'capital' (a commonly employed metaphor) likewise informed thinking about poor relief. On the one hand, the pauper owned only his ability to work and therefore his entire store of wealth consisted of his physical strength. On the other hand, the total of industrious workers in a state constituted its national treasure and a fund which, like capital, was to be mobilized, invested and increased.[8] Christian Wilhelm Hufeland (a major figure in Berlin medical circles) insisted that 'only the sick-man lacks all resources'.[9] Hufeland, therefore, measured the excellence of health care not only in mortality but also in morbidity rates.

If no one disputed the value of a healthy and hard-working population to a state, less like-mindedness existed on how best to promote and preserve it. Agreement on the serious insufficiencies of the hospitals, the almshouses, indeed the whole structure of charity in the eighteenth century, did not automatically create consensus on how their failings might be remedied. Almost everyone admitted that the old leprosaria and *lazarettos* consistently broke down under the new demands now placed on them. Censure of hospitals by physicians and others advocated a whole series of improvements: changes in sickroom and ward design, novel if not particularly practical or efficacious ventilation technologies designed to banish the noxious 'spital air', dismemberment of mammoth institutions, a tighter financial administration, better training for the nursing and surgical staffs, and on. The questioning of hospitals in their extant forms, combined with dissatisfaction with current forms of poor relief, led to a fertile period of experimentation in hospital planning *and* with forms of medical care, especially forms of domiciliary aid, contrived either to supplement hospital care or replace hospitals altogether. Hamburg soon surged to the fore in presenting the world with what was seen as an exemplary form of what domiciliary care could accomplish.[10]

Until the end of the 1760s, Hamburg offered little medical care to the domiciled poor and even less to workers. City magistrates and parish officers could afford temporary assistance in emergencies, but no system for aiding the sick poor on a regular basis existed other than sending them to the ancient plague hospital, the *Pesthof*. These circumstances were occasionally mitigated by the ministrations of individual physicians and surgeons who held special sessions for the poor or treated ophthalmic, dermatological or gynaecological complaints free of charge. Nor should one ignore the probable richness of 'fringe' medicine. Still, it seems safe to argue that the medical care the ordinary labourer received was meagre and probably bad without suggesting that even those who enjoyed excellent care by the standards of the day much benefited from it. The municipality historically had shown far more interest in separating the sick from the well. In the words of a 1714 plague edict, 'the preservation of the city' demanded not only the isolation of the poor, the sick, and the 'miserable' from the rest of human society, but also, especially in times of plague, dictated the 'immediate removal of beggars, begging Jews, and vagabonds'.[11]

By the middle of the eighteenth century, however, perceptions of the labouring poor had merged with new directions in medical education to produce a series of clinics, dispensaries and domiciliary programmes. Ernst Gottfried Baldinger, a Leiden graduate and Boerhaave disciple, founded what was to become the most influential of early clinics at the University of Göttingen in 1773. Many of his students later established similar 'klinische Instituten' at other major universities throughout central and eastern Europe. Baldinger's clinic worked as a school for medical students and an out-patient facility. Patients too ill to be moved were often visited in their homes. This clinic, like others, extended free medical care to at least some part of the labouring classes, although patients tended to be regarded in the first instance as pedagogic raw material.[12]

Baldinger's clinic apparently also sowed the seeds of more daring innovations in medical care. Late in life, he reminisced with pride that 'nine physicians who practise in Hamburg today and who once attended my clinic ... have organized a system of medical care [there] that is admirable in all its details'.[13] The system he so lauded attempted to fill some yawning gaps in the municipality's poor relief structure by organizing domiciliary medical care. Hamburg's domiciliary programmes not only were innovative but also elicited widespread interest and frequent imitation in the closing decades of the century.

In 1768 several physicians in Hamburg volunteered to provide medical care and medicines to the poor for a trial period of two years. This plan (like its successors) was financed through subscription. Despite a promising beginning, however, the enterprise folded within eighteen months. Still, a pattern had been laid down and ten years later, in 1778, many of the same people picked up the strands and founded a second institution, namely the Medical Relief (*Institut für kranke Hausarmen*). It remained active until 1788 when it was incorporated into the newly established General Poor Relief as its Medical Deputation. All three medical charities acknowledged the goals set forth in 1768:

1 'to save the lives and preserve the health of thousands'
2 'to return many upright and honest workers to the state'
3 'to reduce the distress of suffering humanity'.[14]

All three responded to at least some of the sanitary and social problems generated by urbanization and economic growth.

Ultimately the goal of medical relief was the prevention of impoverishment. The plan originally sketched out for the care of the sick poor drew clear connections between disease, illness, accidents and poverty. In calling for contributions, reformers even constructed typical 'case studies'. A father, the sole breadwinner for his wife and several children, falls ill. First he tries a home remedy. When that fails, he hurries to the 'next, best' apothecary or turns to someone who maintains 'I can cure that'. Instead of improving, however, he sinks deeper into illness and destitution. Finally his wife is left a widow, his children, orphans. Then she must carry on alone, as best she can, until she too, worn out by drudgery and worry, follows her husband to the grave. Perhaps she has already buried some of her children, children 'who with better care could have become useful members of the republic'. A different, but just as tragic a fate supposedly awaited such a family when the father did not pass away but remained an invalid, chained to his bed for the rest of his days.[15] The concerns reflected here were political and economic: only healthy persons, not cripples and invalids, were valuable to the state. Medical care for the labouring poor seemed an attractive quick fix for many of the seemingly intractable problems of urban impoverishment. The first published report of the Medical Relief boasted that through its efforts 'many people . . . have regained their health, [people] we can return to the state as more useful and far healthier members [of society] than they were previously, and thus [we] stop up a wellspring of the bitterest want'. At the same time the Medical Relief reduced the burden on other charitable institutions as well as cutting economic loss due to illness. And, according to its advocates, it mobilized resources effectively toward a specific goal, instead of relying on the unreliable and capricious sources of individual charity.[16]

The proponents of medical charity accepted to a large degree structural definitions of poverty. They claimed that illness as well could not be facilely regarded as self-induced for 'illness is an evil of the human condition' and hard labour often caused ill-health. Yet these reformers never totally resolved the conflict between regarding poverty (or illness) as the product of impersonal forces, and seeing these conditions as resulting from individual moral flaws. The Medical Relief, for example, assured its supporters that it did not treat diseases arising from 'criminal dissipations', from imprudence, or from lack of restraint. Read here, not only venereal diseases and alcoholism, but also the pregnancies of unwed mothers.[17] In fact, however, all three medical charities handled such cases and, despite guidelines to the contrary, provided some long-term home-care to invalids and incurables, including those suffering from paresis.[18]

At the same time, the Medical Relief also tried to build a sort of disciplining into its programme. The plainest statement of this is found in the Relief's instructions to its 'beneficiaries'. Briefly summarized, the instructions detailed the conduct of the recipient of aid *vis-à-vis* the Relief; regulating the timing and frequency of visits to physicians, demanding of the patient a 'modest demeanour', threatening termination of support for recalcitrants, denying patients recourse to 'medicines not prescribed by the physicians, whether home-remedies or other quack-medicines', and finally stipulating that 'no one may withdraw from treatment without formally thanking the Relief'.[19] The language sounds officious and unambiguous. However, despite the rhetoric, the disciplinary actions undertaken by the Medical Relief and by its successor, the Medical Deputation of the General Poor Relief, were scattered, mild and few. For example, while the 1781 *Report* recounted that several patients 'because of their intemperance and wanton ruination of their bodies, their decided rebelliousness and coarse behavior toward their physicians, unmindful of all previous warnings' had been 'surrendered up to their fate', the actual number of these in the first six months was only five (of a total of 321 patients). By 1787 the Relief reported that, although it still found occasion to release patients because of 'their perverse nature or because of their unsatisfactory adherence to physicians' orders', such cases were ever less frequent.[20] The evidence suggests that the Relief was far less draconian and uncompromising in its use of force than it might have been. The number of patients who were denied care because they were 'insubordinate' was always tiny and neither the Medical Relief nor the General Poor Relief can be seen as willing and eager collaborators in physicians' bid for a medical monopoly. Doctors themselves were not infrequently reprimanded for unbecoming conduct or the verbal abuse of patients.[21]

More important here than any programme of discipline was the realization that one was now dealing with a 'new' poor for whom the older forms of medical care (as well as the older forms of charity) were obsolete. Older institutions had failed to meet the demands placed on them by modern urban societies. They had equally failed to mobilize resources constructively or to target the best areas for purposeful intervention. The medical care tendered by the Relief was outdoor or domiciliary, rather than institutional and this preference ultimately rested on the perception of the poor as the labouring poor. The stress on outdoor relief underscored the belief that it was now imperative to reintegrate the pauper into the workaday world. As much as possible he or she was to be caught up again in the productive cycle of the economy and not isolated from it as, for example, admittance to the *Pesthof* obviously would do. Moreover, reformers asserted that despite the undeniable worth of charitable institutions such as hospitals 'it is anyway impossible to admit all those who require assistance'.[22] Clearly home-care circumvented the need for expensive hospital buildings, yet it seemed to offer other attractive advantages: the family nursed its own members, mothers could continue to watch over young children, and breadwinners, if not bedridden, might still be able to work a little. Besides these benefits, the outdoor solution could also boast of greater economy and of a more effective employment of limited resources. Mortality ran strikingly lower than in hospitals (at least apparently) and costs were significantly less. During the first two-and-a-half years of its existence (1779–81), the Medical Relief cared for about 3,500 patients at a total cost of 16,000 Marks, or little more than four Marks nine Shillings each.[23]

The debate, hospitals or visiting care, highlights major shifts in attitudes toward health care and poor relief. The supporters of large-scale visiting programmes rejected existing hospitals as fitting centres for the medical treatment of the labouring poor. Only if the poor were 'dispensable' or 'extraneous' could such old-fashioned institutions remain appropriate venues of medical care. As the new poor were not, however, expendable, the antediluvian 'spitals', like archaic methods of poor relief, and eventually like older forms of avuncular or paternalistic government, no longer supplied timely answers to the modern problems either of illness or impoverishment among the labouring classes or of governing a metropolis. Thus the *Pesthof*, like indoor relief in general, won little backing from Hamburg's reformers. The outmoded early modern hospital, sheltering as it did a mis-mixture of the sick, the aged and the insane, was castigated as 'dustbin relief'. It did little to restore the sufferer to health or the impoverished worker to productivity. The spital, like the almshouse, like all such 'primitive' institutions, had over the course of time become unsuitable places for the new labouring classes. All posed life-threatening hazards to the physical, economic, social and moral well-being of thousands.[24]

If we jump ahead into the 1790s for a moment, we uncover further proofs of how decisive the notion of the labouring poor was to prove. This is most obvious in the General Poor Relief's decision to incorporate those who were *not* 'genuine paupers' into its expansive programme of free medical care. These people 'of modest means and resources', while not actually destitute, often found themselves unable to pay for medical consultations or medications.

Without timely medical intervention it was understood that only poverty could issue from their illnesses. Thus the 1788 *Instructions to Relief Officers* specified that free medical care could also pertain to 'those persons who can secure their own livelihoods and require no assistance as long as they retain their health'. The Relief recognized that these needed prompt assistance to rescue them 'from the perils of poverty when smitten with acute or persistent ailments'.[25]

The General Poor Relief consciously (even gratefully) built on the prior experiences of the Medical Relief. One might see the Medical Relief of 1779-88 as the final, full-dress rehearsal for the General Poor Relief: its predecessor and model. By the early 1790s medical relief within the framework of an ambitiously conceived programme of poor relief had developed into a weapon that struck out forcefully at one of the taproots of poverty: physical incapacity. The Relief offered a wide variety of medical assistance, including, but not limited to, free medical consultations with physicians and surgeons, free medicines, trusses and bandages, the help of a midwife in childbirth and free lying-in, as well as special diets and even monetary assistance during illness that could (and often did) exceed normal levels of support. This free medical care, and especially the 'sick-pay', extricated some families from poverty and prevented others from sinking into destitution at least temporarily. The policy implicitly (but never explicitly, of course!) acknowledged the worker's prerogative of health as well as the municipality's duty to provide support and employment. It reached beyond mere alms-giving and punishment and, admittedly timorously, moved into the realm of social security. It also proved an expensive venture.[26]

Yet the concept of expense was always a relative one. The architects of these new departures in poor relief and medical care were never constrained in the breadth of their vision by mere fiscal considerations nor were they miserly in their charity. Nor did they have to be: contributions flowed freely and generously throughout the 1780s and 1790s. Poor relief administrators measured returns on their 'investments' in the coin of social benefits as well as in a harder currency of Marks and Shillings. Despite precise bookkeeping and the meticulous, public accounting of expenditures, all appreciated that the real profits on social investments were incorporeal ones. Those absorbed in the mapping out of social policies ultimately vindicated outlays of time and money by weighing them against the social gains to be won. This same logic sustained make-work schemes, initiated 'unprofitable' enterprises for employing the poor, and stoked a host of improvements in prisons, schools, hospitals and workhouses. The Relief appealed to the public sense of economics, championing at the same time a new type of philanthropy which preserved, however, a very near attachment to the venerable axioms of Christian charity, brotherly love, and duty, and to the Protestant (or not so Protestant) ethics of hard work, temperance, and thrift.

During the halcyon years of the late 1780s and throughout the 1790s, the programme of medical care was vigorously expanded. The General Poor Relief's Medical Deputation handled almost 50,000 cases from 1788–9 through to 1801, and at least another 40,000–50,000 by 1815.[27] The large numbers reflected the extension of medical care to those *not* registered as paupers: the working poor. For the first time (as we have seen) many members of the working classes who were not destitute became eligible for free medical attention. This was identical to the medical assistance enjoyed by the registered pauper, but with few of the disadvantages and little of the opprobrium that clung to being known as a charity case.[28] The numbers of the non-registered poor who applied for free medical care increased rapidly. In 1788–9 there were only 516, about 12 per cent of all patients. By 1792 there were 1,135, or about 30 per cent. Some reformers rejoiced at this expansion. Voght insisted that 'the increase of the non-registered poor treated [by the Relief] clearly shows how very much this programme contributes to the attainment of our ultimate goal: to prevent destitution'. Still, it also gobbled up great sums of money and the members of the Relief's governing council began to feel that perhaps they were being hoodwinked into advancing free medical care to people who did not need it. A period of more stringent control from 1793 to 1795 (which coincided with a brief economic recession in the city) drastically cut the numbers of the non-registered poor who could easily obtain medical assistance. To reduce expenses, the Relief in 1793 introduced a programme of 'half-free' medical care for those who were unable to pay physicians' fees but who could, it was argued, well afford medicines if prescribed at the low rates set in Hamburg's *Paupers' Pharmacopoeia*. It was a short-lived and not very satisfying experiment. The restrictions were totally abolished by 1796 because the Relief feared that they discouraged people who truly required care from seeking it. After 1796 the numbers of the non-registered poor who obtained medical care shot up so steeply that by 1797–8 a full 36.6 per cent of all those receiving medical care from the Relief were not registered paupers. And these numbers continued to climb. Costs, of course, ascended as well, especially after the Relief established a Lying-in Ward in 1796. Yet even when financially hard-pressed the Relief proved extremely unwilling to cut back on medical care for the non-registered poor.[29] Throughout the 1770s, 1780s and 1790s Hamburg's reformers viewed medical care and medical charity as two of the most valuable and cost-effective tools they possessed to combat poverty and forestall impoverishment.

The rise of this new form of medical charity in the last four decades of the eighteenth century was spawned by the broader economic and social changes transforming Hamburg into a modern *Großstadt*. Hamburg had grown into a metropolis where a large percentage of the population (at least 45–50 per cent) was composed of non-citizen members of a working class that owned little more than its labour: a proletariat. The fortunes of this class rested on the successful functioning of an embryonic system of world trade and on the industries that produced for export.

Urbanization was the context of these developments. The growth and the growing wealth of Hamburg had determined, on the one hand, the great need of the working classes and, on the other, the success of the General Poor Relief. Urbanization, like industrialization, has always been a double-edged sword. Fortunately for Hamburg and for its inhabitants, the 1780s and especially the 1790s were years of almost unprecedented and even feverish economic expansion. But these decades were turbulent in other ways as well. The French Revolution and the Revolutionary Wars threw all Europe into turmoil and although Hamburg at first swelled with the spoils drawn from a war-torn world, this was not to last. The period from 1799 to 1814 was a decade-and-a-half of disaster. Catastrophe followed catastrophe. The British blockaded the Elbe, trade ground to a halt, and finally the French occupied Hamburg from 1806 through to 1814. During these years the delicate balance of renewed civic commitment and prosperity that had engendered and sustained the Medical Relief and the General Poor Relief was upset. During the French occupation and even earlier, since 1799, the Relief found itself in distressing circumstances. It jettisoned programme after programme, trying to stay afloat in a sea of troubles. By 1814 it was little more than an alms-giving institution that merely provided minimal medical care. As Hamburg's elites cut back on aid, they also came to question the very bases of poor relief as they had developed since mid-century. In particular, they came to doubt the wisdom of attempts to prevent impoverishment. Now they believed that poor relief should be concerned only with the alleviation of 'true need'. Thus they dished up a far leaner diet of assistance for the registered pauper and condoned little or no support for the non-registered.[30] The Relief that raised itself from the ashes in 1815 was far different from its predecessor: parsimony and social *laissez-faire* had won the day. A new spirit of frugality and even punishment prevailed. The General Poor Relief in 1815 defended its 'penny-pinching' not only on the basis of fiscal integrity, but also on a more theoretical level:

> Must we not fear . . . that we may support too many unworthy persons and that alms too generously given may undercut feelings of self-confidence and sap an ability to rely on one's own strength, qualities which are the proper means of self-preservation for *each* human being?[31]

Partly this shift in position came from the rise of a new generation of leaders during the difficult days of the early 1800s, men who were far less sanguine than their predecessors of the feasibility of attaining social improvement except through a policy of social and economic *laissez-faire* that would eventually re-establish prosperity. But partly it was the failure of an avuncular government, even one bolstered by new ideas and new spurts of civic involvement, to master the problems of urban growth. The Relief now abandoned the position that economic structures or dislocations in the economy, things over which individuals had little influence and even less control, *principally* determined both poverty and prosperity among the lower classes. Most poverty and most illness, the Relief now insisted, sprang directly from the defects of the poor themselves. Thus, after 1815 the Relief predicated its entire programme on the assuagement of existing distress, and repudiated the prevention of poverty as an idle dream and, more tellingly, as a waste of money.

Medical charity was no exception. In the years after 1800, the Relief turned round 180 degrees and moved away from regarding medical care and medical charity as effective ways of preventing poverty, towards seeing them as *creators* of poverty or at least of dependence. Consequently the 'new' Relief reduced the scope of medical care available to paupers and, above all, available to the non-registered poor. In 1814 the Relief commented at length on what it now regarded as the flaws of free medical care, 'flaws' once praised as virtues!

It became customary for any family which did not exactly live in comfort to request free medical care whenever a family member felt the least bit unwell. . . . [and] so the number of the 'ill' multiplied enormously. Soon these same people began to request monetary support [during their illnesses]. Thus many family-fathers whom previously shame had deterred from turning to the Relief and who, despite large families, really did not by right require aid, began begging for assistance. A child fell sick, and the father realized that it only cost him a trip to the Relief Officer to obtain free medical care. Otherwise he would never have thought to seek medical advice for such an ailment. Now he sees it as his duty. A second illness occurs and he immediately requests monetary support. Once he has come to know the Relief Officer, he approaches him once each winter for a bit of help for just a few months 'because of his many children'! Then he seeks a prolongation, and thus we finally have a man as a registered pauper who perhaps would never have become one if he had had to request alms [instead of only medical care] initially.[32]

In 1816 medical relief was reorganized as a semi-independent organ and care for the non-registered poor began to wither.[33] In the following decade the Relief systematically restricted medical care. In 1824 the Relief stipulated that those who benefited from medical care and from medical care alone must submit to the embossing of their possessions with the stamp of the Relief as the registered poor had to do. Likewise, they had to name the Relief as their universal heir.[34]

The question that remains unanswered is why there was such a shift in attitudes toward medical charity in the first two decades of the nineteenth century. The reformers of the second half of the eighteenth century had pursued a vision of civic responsibility and social amelioration that drew on venerable traditions of avuncular and paternalistic government but which also recognized the new realities of urbanization and understood the plight of the labouring poor in this new environment. They responded with a programme that called for renewed civic involvement and which also depended (whether they knew it or not) on thriving economic circumstances. Still, Hamburg in the late eighteenth century was rapidly outrunning the ability of city fathers to govern on a basis of civic commitment and face-to-face techniques. Furthermore, the favourable economic climate of the 1780s and 1790s, which had nurtured the ambitious social and charitable undertakings of these years, and which surely also fed the willingness of men to undertake additional civic duties, had been destroyed by the political and economic upheavals of the first years of the nineteenth century. The successors to the eighteenth-century reformers – the early nineteenth-century liberals – followed the less thorny path of social *laissez-faire*. They simply ignored some of the complexities of governing the sprawling metropolis that now confronted them. They accepted, indeed forged, the liberal maxim in social policies that less was really more. Charity came to be viewed as a matter of essentially private initiative. The number of private charities, and especially of medical charities, founded in the nineteenth century testified to the gulf opening up between the public and private spheres and to the gap estranging state and society. The unwillingness of Hamburg's governing elite to grapple with the problems of social amelioration and to consider government intervention to remedy the deeper problems wrought by urbanization, duties that their forefathers had always acknowledged as a legitimate part of communal responsibilities, accounts in good part for the social disasters Hamburg suffered in the nineteenth century; for the almost total inability of the city's elites to come to grips with the cholera epidemic of 1830; for their ineptitude in dealing with the disorder caused by the Great Fire of 1842; and for the renewed outbreak of cholera in 1892 at a time when sanitary reform had banished the disease from the rest of the Atlantic world. There is here no guarantee that the vanished government of fathers and uncles could have done better: it, too, would almost certainly have foundered. But those who guided Hamburg after 1815 had no better idea of how to cope with the problems of urban and economic gigantism even while they reaped its massive rewards.

Acknowledgement

The author and editors would like to thank Oxford University Press for permission to include in this chapter material that also appears in M. Lindemann, *Patriots and Paupers: Hamburg, 1712–1830*, Oxford, 1990.

NOTES

1 Some of these mistaken beliefs about German history in the eighteenth

century have been partially corrected by J. Sheehan, *German History, 1770–1866*, Oxford, 1989. His book, however, appeared too late for me to make use of it in this chapter. See also H. U. Wehler, *Deutsche Gesellschaftsgeschichte, I: Vom Feudalismus des Alten Reiches bis zur Defensiven Modernisierung der Reformära, 1700–1815*, Munich, 1987.

2 The *Pesthof* was the major hospital. On the general history of hospital development, see D. Jetter, *Geschichte des Hospitals, Vol. 1: Westdeutschland von den Anfängen bis 1850*, Wiesbaden, 1966; A. Imhof, 'Die Funktionen des Krankenhauses in der Stadt des 18. Jahrhunderts', *Zeitschrift für Stadtgeschichte, Stadtsoziologie und Denkmalpflege*, 1977, vol. 4; and specifically on Hamburg, H. Rodegra, *Vom Pesthof zum Allgemeinen Krankenhaus*, Münster, 1977; and 'Krankenhauswesen', Sammelband in Staatsarchiv Hamburg Bibliothek. On Hamburg's development in these years, see H.-D. Loose and W. Jochmann (eds) *Hamburg: Geschichte der Stadt und ihrer Bewohner*, 2 vols, Hamburg, 1982–6, vol. 1; on the working population, see A. Kraus, *Die Unterschichten Hamburgs in der ersten Hälfte des 19. Jahrhunderts*, Stuttgart, 1965; H. Laufenberg, *Hamburg und sein Proletariat im achtzehnten Jahrhundert*, Hamburg, 1910; and A. Herzig, D. Langewiesche and A. Sywotteck (eds) *Arbeiter in Hamburg*, Hamburg, 1983.

3 C. Voght, *Account of the Management of the Poor in Hamburgh since the Year 1788 in a Letter to some Friends of the Poor in Great Britain*, London, 1796, p. 5.

4 Tenon calculated that the mortality in the Hôtel-Dieu exceeded 1:4.5, 'qui surpasse les mortalités connues': J.-R. Tenon, *Mémoires sur les hôpitaux de Paris*, Paris, 1788, pp. 278, 344–5. See also L. S. Greenbaum, '"Measure of Civilization": the hospital thought of Jacques Tenon on the eve of the French Revolution', *Bulletin of the History of Medicine*, 1975, vol. 49, pp. 51–4 and D. Jetter, 'Frankreichs Bemühen um bessere Spitäler', *Sudhoffs Archiv*, 1969, vol. 49, pp. 164–6.

5 W. Conze, 'Vom "Pöbel" zum "Proletariat": Sozialgeschichtliche Voraussetzungen für den Sozialismus in Deutschland', *Vierteljahrschrift für Sozial- und Wirtschaftsgeschichte*, 1954, vol. 41; J. G. Gagliardo, *From Pariah to Patriot: The Changing Image of the German Peasant, 1770–1840*, Lexington, Ky, 1969; and H. C. Payne, *The Philosophes and the People*, New Haven, Conn., 1976.

6 J. G. Büsch, one of the principal figures in poor relief reform in Hamburg and in Europe in the eighteenth century, viewed the emergence of this 'new poor' as the main reason for a reformation of social policies. Büsch, 'Historischer Bericht von dem Gange und fortdauerenden Verfall des Hamburgischen Armenwesens seit der Zeit der Reformation', in Büsch, *Zwei kleine Schriften die im Werk begriffene Verbesserung des Armenwesens in dieser Stadt Hamburg betreffend*, Hamburg, 1784 [unpag.], and Büsch, *Ueber die Ursachen der Verarmung in Nordischen Handelsstädten und die wirksamsten Mittel denselben zu begegnen*, Hamburg, 1785, pp. 17, 42, 48. See also C. Lis and H. Soly, *Poverty and Capitalism in Pre-Industrial Europe*, Brighton, 1979; F. Tennstedt

and C. Sachße, *Geschichte der Armenfürsorge in Deutschland*, Stuttgart, 1980; and J. Gutton, *La Société et les pauvres en Europe, XVIe – XVIIIe siècles*, Paris, 1974.

7 C. G. Hoffmann, 'Ankündigung einer Anstalt für arme Kranke zu Altdorf im Nürnbergischen', *Journal von und für Deutschland*, January 1786, p. 100, and F. X. von Haeberl, *Abhandlung über öffentliche Armen- und Kranken-Pflege*, Munich, 1820, pp. 191–2.

8 For example L. F. B. Lentin, *Beyträge zur ausübenden Arzneywissenschaft*, 3 vols, Leipzig, 1789–1808, vol. 2, p. 17.

9 *Armen-Pharmakopäe entworfen für Berlin nebst der Nachricht von der daselbst errichteten Armenkrankenverpflegungsanstalt*, 2nd edn, Berlin, 1812, p. 3.

10 See 'Krankenhaus' in G. G. Strelin (ed.) *Realwörterbuch für Kameralisten*, 8 vols, Nördlingen, 1783–96; Haeberl, op. cit.; M. Stoll, *Über die Einrichtung der öffentlichen Krankenhäusern*, Vienna, 1788; 'Kranken-Haus' (1789) and 'Medicinal-Anstalten' (1802) in J. G. Krünitz, *Ökonomisch-technologische Encyklopädie*, 242 vols, Berlin, 1773–1858; Greenbaum, op. cit., pp. 47–8; W. H. McMenemey, 'The hospital movement of the eighteenth century and its development', in F. N. L. Poynter (ed.) *The Evolution of Hospitals in Britain*, London, 1964; Jetter, op. cit.; Zachary Cope, 'The history of the dispensary movement', in Poynter (ed.) op. cit.; F. H. Ellis, 'The background of the London Dispensary', *Journal of the History of Medicine and Allied Sciences*, 1965, vol. 20; C. E. Rosenberg, 'Social class and medical care in nineteenth-century America: the rise and fall of the dispensary', *Journal of the History of Medicine and Allied Sciences*, 1974, vol. 29; H. Brüning, 'Soziale Medizin und Gesundheitsfürsorge: Zur Frage der geschichtlichen Entwicklung der Polikliniken', *Das deutsche Gesundheitswesen*, 1952, vol. 7, pp. 1,522–5; E. Heischkel, 'Medizinischer Unterricht im 17. und 18. Jahrhundert im Spiegel von Briefe und Aufzeichnungen', *Deutsche medizinische Rundschau*, 1969, vol. 3, pp. 292–4, and Heischkel, 'Die Poliklinik des 18. Jahrhunderts in Deutschland', *Deutsches medizinisches Journal*, 1954, vol. 5, pp. 223–5.

11 Two 'topographical' works of the late eighteenth century offer much important information on medical and sanitary conditions in Hamburg: J. J. Rambach, *Versuch einer physisch medizinischen Beschreibung von Hamburg*, Hamburg, 1801, and J. L. von Heß, *Hamburg, topographisch, politisch und historisch beschrieben*, 3 vols, Hamburg, 1786–92. 'Etwas über die hamburgische Gesundheitspolizei aus einem Brief eines reisenden Arztes an seinen Freund L. in Thüringen. Hamburg, den 18. Juni 1805', *Hamburg und Altona*, 1805, vol. 4, no. 2, pp. 355–6. The 1714 plague edict is quoted from J. Klefeker, *Sammlung der Hamburgischen Gesetze und Verfassung*, 12 vols, Hamburg, 1765–73, vol. 12, pp. 63–9.

12 E. G. Baldinger, 'Das göttingische klinische Institut, vom 17. May 1773 bis zum letzten März 1792, unter der Aufsicht von E. G. Baldinger, . . .', *Baldingers Neues Magazin*, 1789, vol. 11, p. 100.

13 Ibid.

14 'Nachricht an das Publikum', *Adreß-Comtoir-Nachrichten*, Hamburg, 14 May 1768.

15 *Plan zum Vortheil der hiesigen kranken Haus-Armen*, Hamburg, 1779, paragraph 2, also in *Adreß-Comtoir-Nachrichten*, 20 and 27 May 1779.

16 *Nachricht von der neuerrichteten medicinischen Anstalt für kranken Haus-Arme in Hamburg* (hereafter *Nachricht 1781*), Hamburg, 1781, pp. 16, 20, and *Zweite Sammlung der Nachrichten vom medicinischen Armen-Institut in Hamburg. Vom 1sten Jul. 1781 bis Januar 1784* (hereafter *Nachricht 1784*), Hamburg, 1784, p. 40.

17 *Nachricht 1781*, p. 20.

18 See especially the regular reports on the activities of the Medical Deputation in each issue of *Nachrichten von der Einrichtung und dem Fortgang der Hamburgischen Armen-Anstalt*, nos 1–54 (1788–1840) and on the treatment of incurables, Staatsarchiv Hamburg (hereafter StAHbg), Allgemeine Armenenstalt I (hereafter AAI), 107.

19 'Verhaltungs-Regeln für diejenigen, welche vom Armen-Institut curirt seyn wollen' (May 1779) in *Nachricht 1781*, pp. 10–12. See also the similar regulations insisted on by the Medical Deputation of the General Poor Relief. Paragraphs 16–17, 4, 6–7, and 14 of 'Verhaltungs-Regeln für die auf Kosten der Armen-Anstalt zu verpflegenden Kranken und deren Angehörigen', reprinted in J. A. Günther, *Ueber die Einrichtung der mit der Hamburgischen allgemeinen Armenanstalt verbundenen Kranken-Besuch-Anstalt*, Leipzig, 1793, pp. 3–13.

20 The *Nachricht 1781* (reporting on the period 1 July 1779 through 1 January 1780) and 'Nachricht von dem Fortgang des medicinischen Armen-Instituts in der lezten Hälfte des Jahrs 1787', *Adreß-Comtoir-Nachrichten*, 4 February 1788.

21 See for example StAHbg, AAI, 99, 'Die Armenärzte – Anstellung, Beschwerden –, 1784–1792, 1823–1844'.

22 D. Nootnagel, *Briefe eines Arztes*, Hamburg, 1777, p. 288.

23 *Nachricht 1781*, p. 29, and *Nachricht 1784*, p. 44. F. B. Weber, *Staatswissenschaftlicher Versuch über das Armenwesen und die Armenpolizey mit vorzüglicher Hinsicht auf die dahin eingeschlagende Literatur*, Göttingen, 1807, pp. 184–6, also commented on the economy of the Hamburg system. The average per patient cost was low (in 1801 only 4 Marks 1 Shilling) and, he pointed out, 'similar treatment in the hospitals there costs at least twice as much'.

24 The debate over which offered more advantages – domiciliary care or hospitals – took place throughout Europe. See the summary of the debate in Krünitz, op. cit., the articles on 'Kranken-Haus' and 'Medicinal-Anstalten'. Among the most prolific advocates of domiciliary care were two Hamburgers: Johann Arnold Günther, a wealthy merchant and later Senator in Hamburg, and the physician, Daniel Nootnagel. See Günther, *Argumente und Erfahrungen über Kranken-Besuch-Anstalten aus den 2jährigen Rechnungs Abschlüßen des Medicinal Departments der Hamburgischen Armenanstalt*, Hamburg, 1791; Günther, 'Kranken-besuch Anstalten in Hamburg', *Staats Anzeiger*, 1791, vol. 16, pp. 163–7; Günther, 1793, op. cit.; Günther, 'Vorarbeiten zur Revision der hamburgischen Medizinal-Polizei, auf Veranlassung des im Jahr 1796, erledigten Physikats und Subphysikats, vom Senator Günther in Hamburg', *Beyträge zum Scherfs Archiv*, 1798, vol. 7, no. 2; and by

Nootnagel, 'Über Krankenanstalten, Vortheile der Kranken Besuch Anstalt', *Staats Anzeiger*, 1785, vol. 7; and his *Briefe*, passim. See also 'Antrag der Medicinal Deputation, 1789', StAHbg, AAI, 106; *Nachricht 1781*, pp. 20–2; 'Convention zwischen der Armen-Anstalt und dem Pesthof. Vom Jahr 1789'; 'Extractus Protocolli der Medicinal-Deputation', 14 January 1789, StAHbg, AAI, 105.

25 Quote from paragraph 50 of 'Des großen Armen Collegii nähere Erläuterung für die Herrn Armen-Pfleger. Im August 1788', *Vollständige Einrichtungen der neuen Hamburgischen Armenanstalt*, Hamburg, 1788, pp. 98–100.

26 On the programme and goals of medical relief, see Günther, 1793, op. cit.; *6te Nachricht* (June 1790), p. 56; *9te Nachricht* (March 1791), pp. 85–108; on types of care offered, *15te Nachricht* (February 1794), pp. 222–3 and *24te Nachricht* (September 1798), pp. 131. See also the deliberations of the Medical Deputation from 1788 to 1806 in StAHbg, AAI, 109.

27 Number of patients treated by the General Poor Relief: 1788–9, 4,226; 1789–90, 4,269; 1790–1, 4,474; 1791–2, 4,018; 1792–3, 3,264; 1793–4, 3,424; 1794–5, 3,569; 1795–6, 3,339; 1796–7, 3,045; 1797–8, 3,175; 1798–9, 3,379, *1799–1800 (*a change in the method of accounting necessitated a 'long' year here running from 1 October 1799 to 30 December 1800), 3,545; and 1801, 4,738. Total number of patients treated in the period 1788–1801: 48,465. Sources: *21te Nachricht* (February 1797), p. 67; *23te Nachricht* (January 1798), p. 112; *25te Nachricht* (July 1799), p. 170; *27te Nachricht* (February 1800), p. 234; *28te Nachricht* (January 1801), p. 273; and *30te Nachricht* (May 1803), pp. 342–3.

28 See note 25.

29 See StAHbg, AAI, 106; *14te Nachricht* (May 1793), pp. 207–8; *22te Nachricht* (June 1797), pp. 85–6; and the deliberations of the Medical Deputation especially in the years 1793 and 1796, StAHbg, AAI, 94. See also 'Ersparungs- und Verbesserungsvorschläge betr. die Armenkrankenpflege und die Bekanntmachung über die Aufnahme halbfreier Kranker, 1789–1793'.

30 On the general conditions of assistance, see 'Bericht der von dem großen Armen-Collegio, um Vorschläge über die Wiederherstellung der Armen-Anstalt und die Modalität ihres künftigen Bestandes zumachen, Niedergesetzten Commission, abgestattet in dem Collegio den 27sten Juny 1814'; 'Nachricht an die Herren Armen-Pfleger über den Geschaftsgang bei der Armenfürsorge', in C. D. Anderson and J. M. Lappenberg (eds) *Sammlung der Verordnungen der freien Hanse-Stadt Hamburg seit deren Wiederbefreiung im Jahre 1814*, 10 vols, Hamburg, 1815–29, vol. 2, pp. 265–330; and *37te Nachricht* (October 1816), pp. 254–5. On the retreat from the belief that economic conditions triggered most instances of poverty, see *38te Nachricht* (July 1818), p. 258 and also Caspar Voght, *Gesammeltes aus der Geschichte der Hamburgischen Armenanstalt während ihrer fünfzigjährigen Dauer*, Hamburg, 1834, p. 114.

31 *37te Nachricht* (October 1816), p. 254.

32 Quoted in Werner von Melle, *Die Entwicklung des öffentlichen Armen-*

wesens in Hamburg, Hamburg, 1883, pp. 141–2.

33 'Rat- und Bürgerschluß, das Institut für die Heilung kranken Armen betreffend', 22 August 1816, in Anderson and Lappenberg, op. cit., vol. 3, pp. 137–52, and 'Verordnung des Instituts für die Heilung kranker Armen', in ibid., pp. 152–87. Relief Officers still, however, participated in the provision of medical care, although their competencies and freedom of action were now considerably restricted. See 'Nachricht an die Herren Armenpfleger' (1817), in ibid., vol. 4, pp. 310–27.

34 Von Melle, op. cit., p. 144.

8

THE COSTS AND BENEFITS OF CARING

Nursing charities, c.1830–c.1860

Anne Summers

The rise of the movement for nursing reform in Britain has often been depicted as a sub-plot in the larger history of the voluntary hospitals. Accounts of the career of Florence Nightingale – with which most references to nursing history still begin and end – focus on her visits to hospitals, her interest in the rationalization of ward work, her studies of ventilation and drainage, and her overriding concern with the management of the environment of the (predominantly institutionalized) patient.[1] There has also been speculation that, well before the outbreak of the Crimean War, the advances in surgical technique and the more specialized medical treatment pioneered in the voluntary hospitals led surgeons and physicians to demand a better qualified class of auxiliary helpers.[2] On either count, changes in nursing have been seen as the outcome of changes in the nature of voluntary hospital provision for the sick poor; inasmuch as nursing has been characterized as a philanthropic activity it has been by virtue of its relationship with these particular institutional medical charities.

This chapter will, by contrast, focus as much on nursing in the domiciliary sector as in the hospitals in the mid-nineteenth century. The records of two nursing charities, the Institution for Nursing Sisters founded by Elizabeth Fry in 1840, and the Training Institution for Nurses, St John's House, founded by high church Anglicans in 1848, offer a particularly fruitful source for the study of the relationship between domiciliary, institutional, philanthropic and commercial medical provision in this period. These sources, and evidence on the activities of religious visiting societies, demonstrate that nursing provision and reform had, in the first half of the century, a largely autonomous history: a rationale and a momentum which evolved separately from, and sometimes ran counter to, developments in the voluntary hospital sector. If there is, indeed, a text to which nursing history forms a sub-plot it is the history of Victorian Christianity. Paradoxically, perhaps, this line of inquiry has the unexpected result of throwing light on both clinical and non-clinical aspects of hospital development that would not have been provided by a hospital-centred method of research.

It is a truth universally acknowledged among medical historians, but not always made explicit in their publications, that for much of the nineteenth century neither minor nor major illness was automatically thought to require institutional treatment. The rich, and indeed any patients with pretensions to gentility, were nursed at home; the poor did everything in their power to avoid entering the workhouse infirmary or sick ward. The voluntary hospitals catered for a small section of the sick population – the deserving poor bearing letters of recommendation from subscribers. Moreover, they did not treat many serious conditions such as tuberculosis, cancer, smallpox and other fevers, and venereal disease; they rarely treated illness in small children, and did not deliver babies. Over time, the rules of some of these hospitals were modified, and specialist hospitals were established for a number of the excluded conditions.[3] But, over most of Britain, most sickness was treated at home. It is, therefore, a more than plausible assumption that those members of the charitable classes who were in closest touch with the medical needs of the sick poor were not those who founded and governed their hospitals, but those who visited them in their homes.

Clergymen, medical men and many benevolent men and women found informal ways to visit and help their less fortunate neighbours in the early years of the nineteenth century. However, the most important initiatives in formalizing such practices were made by the District Visiting Societies of the established and dissenting churches.[4] These distributed spiritual, material and medical comforts to the homes of the poor. (It is, indeed, due to the pervasiveness of their work and organization that the term 'district nursing' is used in Britain to describe non-commercial domiciliary nursing care.) District visiting was in many ways an attempt to re-create the social relations of the rural parish in a period of rapid urbanization. Preaching in 1830 on the occasion of the formation of a Provident District Society in Liverpool, the Rev. J. Aspinall affirmed that in the country it was unnecessary to construct social links between the classes, as these arose quite naturally:

when, however, men crowd and herd together, the very force of circumstances is opposed to the existence of the brotherly love recommended by the Apostle; . . . As the multitude swells into thousands, tens of thousands, or hundreds of thousands, the lines of demarcation between the different orders and classes of society are more and more widened.[5]

So, just as the rural vicar or his wife kept a stock of medicines or baby linen to help out poorer parishioners in crisis, a District Visiting Society such as that in Brighton thought it appropriate in 1827 to sponsor a dispensary, and to encourage 'private medical men' to 'visit the poor more extensively'.[6]

Nursing and medical provision was a channel of philanthropy which, from the point of view of the giver, had many advantages. Visitors were aware that their attempts to improve the domestic and financial habits of the poor were often resented; on the other hand, they felt that to give charitable help without further inquiry or advice merely encouraged scrounging and dependency. However, since a 'deserving' family might sink into long-term pauperism through the illness and unemployment of its wage-earners, medical assistance had the saving merit of being a preventive and enabling measure. It is to be noted in this context that even the harsh provisions of the New Poor Law did not oblige those seeking medical relief to submit to the 'workhouse test': sick paupers received medical attendance or extra rations on an 'outdoor' basis, in their own homes. For the pastorally minded, the sick – and death-beds of the poor had the added 'attraction' of offering opportunities for religious conversion and general family edification. As 'A Country Clergyman' summed it up in 1826:

When disease assails the abode of such poverty, a more *legitimate* subject of sympathy and commiseration is afforded to the visitor, and the poor man's spirit that would revolt from the language of admonition and reproof, is in a great degree quelled; his personal fears, or his natural affections, interpose their softening power, and thus a fitter occasion for influencing the heart occurs on the one hand, and a greater readiness to receive the Christian influence exists on the other. (original emphasis)[7]

Significantly this passage is taken from a pamphlet entitled *Protestant Sisters of Charity; A letter addressed to the Lord Bishop of London*

Developing a Plan for Improving the Arrangements at present existing for Administering Medical Advice and Visiting the Sick Poor. The pastoral opportunities afforded by nursing the poor lay behind much of the growing interest in reviving sisterhoods within the Protestant churches in this period. In his *Colloquies,* published in 1829, the poet laureate Robert Southey envisaged a sisterhood which, while working primarily in hospitals, would also 'lessen the pressure upon them by seeking out the sick, and attending them in their own habitations'.[8] The first practical initiative in this direction was taken soon afterwards by one of his correspondents, a Lancashire clergyman named Joshua Hornby. In 1829 Hornby founded an association in Liverpool, which set up a nurses' home under a female superintendent; after its inmates had spent a short period working in hospital under supervision, they were sent out to the homes of the poor. The experiment, for reasons which will be explained below, was short-lived.[9]

The outbreak of the cholera epidemic of 1831–2 may have prompted further consideration of the nursing needs of the poor. The Rev. John Henry Newman's mother wrote to him with a scheme which suggested a knowledge of the Liverpool experiment:

> Should it [the cholera epidemic] increase, I wish you could have that cottage in Littlemore for headquarters for nurses to be on the spot, without mixing with uncontaminated families, and for a depot of medicines, etc. And I should think it a privilege, while health permits, for you to consider me *head nurse.* I have the whole in my head, should it be ordained that our vicinity is to suffer under the visitation.

This plan does not appear to have materialized: in Oxford as elsewhere at this date, home and hospital nursing of cholera victims was organized by the local Board of Health.[10]

The first sustained attempt to create a nursing service for the poor along these lines had to wait until 1840, when Elizabeth Fry founded her Institution for Nursing Sisters in Bishopsgate, London. Throughout the intervening decade she had been a central figure in the discussion of visiting and nursing schemes. Southey had in 1829 proposed that she and her collaborator Amelia Opie should take a leading part in a nursing sisterhood: Elizabeth told her friend that 'I have seen the thing wanted to be done, ever since the days of my youth. . . . I think that what has been accomplished in Liverpool is very important'. Her connection with Liverpool visiting circles is also evidenced by Aspinall's comment that the idea of the Liverpool Provident District Society 'emanated' from her, and that a meeting had been convened 'to take her views of the matter into consideration, and a Committee appointed to organise and digest such a plan as might seem best calculated to carry them into effect'.[11]

After Hornby's nursing experiment ground to a halt, Mrs Fry drew fresh inspiration from developments in Germany. Pastor Theodore Fliedner, who had himself in 1823 been inspired by her example to undertake missions to prisoners, in 1837 established at Kaiserswerth on the Rhine an Institution for Deaconesses, who worked as nurses and teachers. In 1840 Mrs Fry visited him there, and returned to England fired by his example.[12] The ecumenical character of the movement for nursing reform, from High Anglicanism through to the Society of Friends, is certainly one of its most striking features, and seems to have been mirrored by a pattern of common concerns in the visiting movement as a whole.[13] When, in 1848, Elizabeth Fry's initiative was followed by the foundation of a High Anglican nursing institution, St John's House, sectarian differences were apparent in the constitution of each sisterhood, but their working practices were remarkably similar.[14]

Both the Fry sisters and St John's House (I shall not quote their full titles because these were so alike that they confused even contemporaries) provided free nursing in the homes of the poor; they also functioned as commercial agencies for private nursing. Each supplied their nurses with a uniform, and provided a communal home where they lived, under supervision, in between assignments. A period of between one and three months' probationary training in a voluntary hospital was required before a nurse was admitted as a full member of the sisterhood; she was then guaranteed a salary, full board and free care during sickness. An important 'selling point' for each organization was the provision of trustworthy character references for the nurses sent on private cases. The Fry sisters had to be Protestants, and all written testimonials were personally followed up by a member of the all-female committee of management before probationers were admitted. St John's House sisters and nurses had to be members of the Church of England, with appropriate clerical recommendations. After admission, checks were maintained on the nursing staff by the requirement of written reports from home patients, or from their families or friends.

St John's House had, beyond its mission to the poor, the general aim of winning approval for the (allegedly 'Romanizing') movement towards establishing sisterhoods within the Church of England. It set itself the further task of raising the character of nurses generally through close religious supervision: this was to be achieved through the appointment of a clerical Master of the House, and by the recruitment of ladies as unpaid sisters, who would set the nurses 'the example of persons in a higher position undertaking these duties out of pure religion and charity'.[15] The Fry Institution appointed a home superintendent of the same social class as the nurses, and dropped the title 'Protestant Sisters of Charity' in 1841, out of deference to low church opinion.[16] From the outset, hospitals and other institutions applied to both agencies for supernumerary nurses and supervisory staff, as well as for general advice. The Fry sisters worked in many London and provincial hospitals, and in some provincial workhouse infirmaries between 1841 and 1849; St John's House supplied nurses to London hospitals and was consulted over plans for nursing reorganization, for example by the London Fever Hospital in 1857, and by the United Hospital, Bath, in 1861.[17]

Once the nursing sisterhoods had become widely accepted as a reliable source of labour, their champions could advance larger claims for them, and with greater confidence than would have been possible in Southey's day. In an endeavour which matched that of the Visiting Societies to bring the ever-growing urban masses within the reach of parish organization, sisterhoods were pictured as vital weapons in the battle to recover hospitals for the established church. The voluntary hospitals had been conceived within a framework of Anglican charity and ministry, as is shown by the appointment of chaplains and the requirement that discharged patients should give thanks for recovery at their parish church. As patient numbers grew, and as the teaching functions of the hospitals expanded, it was perhaps inevitable that less importance should be attached to pastoral care.

In 1854 a little book entitled *Hospitals and Sisterhoods* was published by Mary Stanley, who at the end of that year helped Florence Nightingale to recruit her first contingent of war nurses, and herself brought a second contingent out to Scutari.[18] Mary Stanley quoted with approval an unnamed former London hospital chaplain for whom the wards provided not only a captive audience for the gospels, but also a living sermon on the physical consequences of sin, and on the nearness of death and the soul's final reckoning. He concluded:

If then we desire to benefit the poor; if we would diffuse the blessed influences of religion amongst the lower orders of society; if we would reclaim citizens to our country, and children to our God, let us watch with anxious care over the Hospitals of our land. Let it be our concern to procure for them the blessings of our pure Reformed religion, and to defend them from the baneful influence of lukewarmness on the one hand, and of error upon the other.[19]

For such clergymen, there was great appeal in the prospect of reinforcing the chaplain's work with the ministry of godly women; it was thought that only the sisterhoods could systematically supply such a class of nurses. (In passing, it may be remarked that some writers considered it an equally urgent matter to save medical students from the corrupting attentions of less pious nurses.)[20] Where the sisterhood 'party' had sympathizers on hospital boards of management, it could help to sway the decision to invite the sisterhoods on to the wards. In 1856 King's College Hospital, London, contracted out its nursing and domestic arrangements to St John's House for a fixed annual sum. King's example was followed in 1866 by Charing Cross Hospital, London. At the time the Rev. R. Few, who was a governor both of St John's House and of Charing Cross, chaired the hospital's sub-committee on nursing reorganization and flatly refused to consider a secular model for change.[21] Another Charing Cross governor at the time was John Archibald Shaw Stewart, an active member of the high church movement; he was also a governor of St George's, Guy's and Middlesex Hospitals.[22] (In 1861 his sister, Jane, taking on the superintendence of the first official female army nursing service, had extracted from the War Office the condition that all her nurses should be Anglicans, a religious bar that obtained nowhere else in the army.)[23] 'Graduates' of the sisterhoods were often favoured candidates as matrons or lady superintendents: the Middlesex appointed Godiva Miriam Thorold, formerly of All Saints', in 1870; Leicester Royal Infirmary appointed Margaret Elizabeth Burt, ex-St John's, in 1875, and Miss Burt's move to Guy's in 1879 provoked a celebrated crisis over the role of educated ladies in hospital nursing.[24] Although the sisterhood movement continued to arouse controversy, there is little doubt that until the early 1870s, when the Nightingale Training School began to produce a strong cohort of 'graduates' of its own, the sisterhoods in practical terms exercised the most widespread influence in the movement for nursing reform, both within and outside the hospitals.[25]

What this account suggests is that initiatives to alter the nursing arrangements of hospitals came not only from outside the hospitals themselves, but also from outside the realm of medicine. The suppliers of nursing services to the poor had criticisms to make of existing facilities which were dictated by religious priorities, and which were not a response to demands from either the medical profession or from patients. However, a closer study of the *clinical* histories of the Fry Institution and St John's House produces a more complex narrative of the relation between supply and demand than this. It also brings us back to a focus on the care of the sick in their own homes. And it is at this point that it is appropriate to return to Hornby's experiment of 1829, and to ask why it failed.

In its preamble, Hornby's association stated:

> The poor are entirely without professed Nurses; even the rich are, in many instances, consigned to the negligence of an ignorant or unfeeling Nurse. The amount of misery which is thus occasioned is such as would astonish, if it were known.[26]

By 1831 the association was departing from what its founder considered to be its original ethos. Hornby and his colleague Adam Hodgson resigned on the grounds that 'as soon as it appeared that they were educating a valuable class of persons, it was sought to make them available to the upper classes as monthly nurses'.[27]

In the 1840s the nursing needs of the rich were to have less destructive consequences for the Fry Institution and St John's House; but they were nevertheless to exercise a profound and unanticipated effect on the development of each. In deciding to undertake fee-paying work, both institutions intended to subsidize their charitable nursing, and to put themselves on such a sound financial footing that their missions to the poor could be expanded. However, financial considerations could lead to contradictory policies: for example the potentially benevolent were encouraged to subscribe by the offer of priority treatment in their own applications for nursing assistance. Keeping afloat was an endless struggle. There were slack seasons when there was little demand for nurses, but salaries had still to be paid – as they also did when, as frequently happened in busy seasons, the nurses fell ill and were again unable to bring any income into the institution. Not every genteel client, moreover, could afford the full fee of a guinea per week, and the institutions often had to be satisfied with less.

St John's House, where the sisters were unsalaried, should in principle have been better able to weather financial storms and continue to provide for the poor. But the number of sisters was not more than four or five at most in the early years. In 1850 the Lady Superintendent expressed her concern over a growing preoccupation with the profit motive: 'Nor does it seem well to refuse a nurse when the means of the party make the full payment impossible lest money getting, not charity, be considered the principle of the Institution'.[28]

Matters were not helped in 1852 when it emerged that the House's accountant had been embezzling funds and that the Master himself was implicated in the deception.[29] In these circumstances it was inevitable that the home nursing needs of the poor, which were labour-intensive and unprofitable, should be given low priority. The entry in the minutes of the Fry Institution's committee of management of 26 October 1849, that henceforth one or two nurses should be employed exclusively for the poor, suggests that here too the anomaly had become painfully obvious.[30]

In meeting the demand for the home nursing of the rich or genteel, were these institutions utterly subverting their original charitable purposes? The rationing of staff and time available to the homes of the poor would certainly suggest so, and there is other evidence to support this conclusion. The rich, as has often been said, are different from the poor: they have more money. Rich patients offered their nurses a clean working environment, where other servants took care of the domestic chores. They might give their nurses presents when they left.[31] Working conditions among poor patients offered a disagreeable contrast, and some nurses took no pains to hide feelings of resentment or even contempt in their management of 'poor cases'.

In 1844 a report on Hannah Cornish, one of the Fry sisters, stated that 'the self importance acquired by nursing in very high and wealthy families makes the Sisters either uncomfortable or unpleasant with persons in less affluent circumstances'. Three years earlier, a report on a Mary Ann Cordingly had concluded:

I must say that the poor old lady she attended did not think her manner considerate or gentle. My own opinion is that her visits should be confined to the houses of the wealthy and that she should never be sent to nurse such a poor family.[32]

In 1845 Jane Ann Medwinter was 'reproved for making a difficulty of attending a poor case and returning suddenly from it', and it was considered worthy of remark that a candidate for membership of the Fry Institution, a shoemaker's widow who was the daughter of a baker, 'has no objection to poor cases'.[33]

Despite these departures from the pious spirit in which the Institution had been founded, the nursing sisters' experience among fee-paying clients did have positive implications where the care of the poor was concerned. Moving as they did between the hospitals (where they received probationary training and undertook supernumerary ward work) and the homes of the prosperous, the sisters found much to criticize in the standards of institutional care. In 1842 some of the Fry sisters who were temporarily engaged at the London Hospital threatened to leave because it was so dirty.[34] In 1849 the Lady Superintendent of St John's House considered that the hospitals were not providing enough instruction in preparing 'little delacacies [sic] which are so necessary for the sick'. She yearned for a 'Sanitorium' [sic] to be attached to the House so that the probationers could learn 'much that cannot be taught at Hospitals which it is necessary they should learn before they can be very efficient as private Nurses in the higher ranks of life'.[35] And in 1851 the medical men on the Council of St John's House were asked to find out 'whether some arrangement may not be made at the Hospitals for giving probationers better instruction as to night duty'.[36]

This last was a significant request. Over and over again, in reading hospital records or published histories, one is struck by the meagre provision made for night nursing, even where some reforms took place in daytime arrangements. In private practice there was no question of drafting in a class of inferior, lower-paid 'watchers' for night duty. The same nurse was on call throughout an assignment, and if she became too fatigued, another nurse replaced her. By 1851 the Fry Institute was asking that 'if possible' a nurse should be 'allowed' to rest every third night on a case.[37] By 1865 St John's also stipulated that a nurse should not sit up more than two consecutive nights, unless she had been permitted six hours' rest outside the sick-room during the day.[38] Another area where the domiciliary position of sole responsibility brought higher standards was in surgical nursing. Most hospitals employed dressers and clinical clerks for the bulk of their surgical nursing up to the 1870s and beyond.[39] But operations were performed in wealthy patients' homes with a nurse in attendance, and she remained in charge of post-operative care.[40] The St John's House records suggest that some nurses may have specialized in this field, such as Marianne Wright. The latter's first case was a surgical one; she was later recommended for being 'particularly nice and skilful in her management of the wound', and subsequently attended mainly surgical cases, including one of cataract, until her dismissal in 1857 for the misdemeanour of a secret marriage.[41]

Thus, when the nurse who was highly experienced in private care among the wealthy entered hospital service or, indeed, hospital supervision, her arrival was attended with many advantages for the institutionalized poor: higher standards of cleanliness and invalid cookery; higher standards of surgical skill and knowledge; higher standards of night watching. When hospitals began to contract out their nursing to the sisterhoods, as King's College and Charing Cross did to St John's House in 1856 and 1866, and as University College Hospital, London, did to All Saints' in 1862, the impact of these different standards was, of course, more marked. There was, indeed, something of a clash of expectations between sisters and governors. Initial opposition to contracting out domestic and nursing work to the sisterhoods had been motivated by fears of 'Romanizing' proselytization; after the sisterhoods were installed, there was unexpected controversy over financial issues. Significantly these related to the costs of diet and hygiene.

After the installation of St John's House at Charing Cross in 1866, the Financial Committee drew attention to 'the extraordinary increase in the consumption of articles of food etc., especially Wine, Brandy, Bottled Porter, Fish and Eggs' and to 'the large consumption of calico used for bandaging'.[42] By 1874 it was generally claimed that sisterhood nursing raised costs per hospital bed, because cleaning work was always separated from nursing proper, necessitating the employment of a larger group of 'scrubbers', and because patients were being fed above their station:

> To a lady, the ordinary diet of a hospital looks plain and uninviting; she forgets that it is probably luxurious in comparison to that which the patient has previously been accustomed; if the latter show any want of appetite, the sister is only too fertile in suggesting delicacies, and, when once 'extras' are introduced, it needs most constant watchfulness to prevent their becoming general. The poor are so well acquainted with the ill effects of a deficiency of food that they over-estimate the

therapeutic advantages of plenty; and the amount of suffering due to dyspepsia from over-eating, to which a surgical patient, backed by a zealous sister, will uncomplainingly submit, under the idea that he is doing himself good, is truly surprising.[43]

It has often been claimed that the poor inmates of the voluntary hospitals paid the human and physical costs of medical and surgical advance for the population as a whole. Treatments applied experimentally to the bodies of the poor were not, until perfected, applied to those of the rich.[44] But the history of the sisterhoods presents a complete reversal of this sequence. Standards developed in the homes of the prosperous made their way into the voluntary hospitals. The stream of benevolence which launched the sisterhoods may have been diverted by commercial considerations away from the *homes* of the poor; but it was re-routed to the *institutions* where they were treated. Those classes of patients who had originally been targeted for pastoral reclamation and a mission of social reconciliation reaped instead an unexpected harvest of clean sheets and bandages, and meals that were too good for them.

This brief sketch suggests that most chronologies of nursing reform are in need of drastic reappraisal. It was not the increasing sophistication of medical and surgical procedures which led to the call for better trained and disciplined nursing staff, but the perception of the urban poor as beings in need of spiritual ministry. Nursing sisterhoods sent their members to hospitals to gain experience of a large variety of cases in the space of a few weeks; not because the hospitals themselves set standards of excellence. It was in the homes of the rich, rather than the hospitals of the poor, that the demand for higher technical standards of sick nursing emerged. Both the religious nursing mission to the poor and the demand for improved nursing among the rich were in evidence by the 1830s; and hospitals had begun to appreciate the merits of sisterhood practice a decade before the outbreak of the Crimean War.

The sisterhoods assured their institutional clientele a sober, respectable, reliable labour force; private patients were promised skill and discretion. Kindness and religious consolation were seen as essential qualities in the sick-room, even if not every nurse was gifted in this respect. Nowhere were such qualities considered alternatives to cleanliness, stamina, medical knowledge and physical dexterity. Religious and clinical imperatives do not appear to have come into conflict, although both Pastor Fliedner and Mrs Fry's daughters criticized her institution for not insisting that 'love to souls should be the leading, compassion to the suffering body the secondary, motive for action'.[45] Those St John's sisters who were obliged to leave King's College Hospital in 1868 in the wake of sectarian controversy were not accused of physically neglecting their patients.[46] Both sisterhoods demonstrated the financial difficulties lying in the way of any systematic attempt to provide home nursing for the poor; St John's 'failures' in this respect drove them to the relative financial security of permanent hospital contracts, and an era of new 'successes'; a similar failure on the part of all other providing agencies contributed to the crisis of overcrowding perceived in the metropolitan hospitals and workhouses in the 1860s.[47]

Because our reading of medical history takes the expansion of the hospital system for granted – together with the development of hospital 'in-house' nurse training schools – the origins of nursing reform in Britain have tended to be obscured. We have 'read back' narrative themes from a familiar social landscape: experimentation, secularization, modernization, professionalization. None of these concepts is adequate to describe a movement which was fed by the desire to spread the Christian faith and to preach a gospel of reconciliation; which, generating missions to the poor, financed and all but subsumed them in services purveyed to the middle and upper classes; and which found its way to the voluntary hospitals by a combination of sectarian fervour and financial embarrassment. The way the story ends is so at variance with the way it begins that we are overwhelmed by the urge to revise it; we cast around for some convenient, rational, organizing principle. Hitherto such principles have been found in the history of the hospital and the biography of Florence Nightingale. It is to be hoped that a new theme such as 'charity' will permit us to re-enter the productive chaos of an unknown past.

Acknowledgements

The research for this chapter was financed by a Fellowship from the Wellcome Trust, which is gratefully acknowledged. The author's colleagues at the Wellcome Unit for the History of Medicine,

145

University of Oxford, gave invaluable support and advice while this work was in progress, but must not be held responsible for its faults and conclusions.

NOTES

1 See for example C. E. Rosenberg, 'Florence Nightingale on contagion: the hospital as moral universe', in Rosenberg (ed.) *Healing and History*, New York, 1979. The most recent work of Nightingale scholarship, M. E. Baly's *Florence Nightingale and the Nursing Legacy*, London, 1986, contains a chapter on district nursing.

2 B. Abel-Smith, *The Hospitals 1800–1948*, London, 1964, pp. 43–5; M. J. Peterson, *The Medical Profession in Mid-Victorian London*, Berkeley, Calif., 1978, pp. 14–15.

3 J. Woodward, *To Do the Sick No Harm*, London, 1974, pp. 45–55; Abel-Smith, op. cit., pp. 22–8; E. G. Thomas, 'The old Poor Law and medicine', *Medical History*, 1980, vol. 24, p. 3.

4 H. D. Rack, 'Domestic visitation: a chapter in early nineteenth-century evangelism', *Journal of Ecclesiastical History*, 1973, vol. 24; D.M. Lewis, 'The evangelical mission to the British working class: a study of the growth of Anglican support for a pan-evangelical approach to evangelism, with special reference to London 1828–60', D.Phil thesis, University of Oxford, 1981. I am indebted to Dr John Walsh for directing me to these sources.

5 Rev. J. Aspinall, *A Sermon preached at St. Michael's Church, Liverpool, 4 April 1830, upon the subject of the Provident District Society now forming in that Town*, Liverpool, 1830, pp. 7–8.

6 *Hints to a Clergyman's Wife*, London, 1832, pp. 79, 80n.; *Hints on District Visiting Societies*, London, 1836, pp. 31, 56.

7 'A Country Clergyman' [Alexander R. C. Dallas], *Protestant Sisters of Charity; A letter addressed to the Lord Bishop of London Developing a Plan for Improving the Arrangements at present existing for Administering Medical Advice and Visiting the Sick Poor*, London, 1826, pp. 9–10. For a later statement of the importance of medical relief in keeping families from degradation and dependency, see E. H. Sieveking, *The Training Institutions for Nurses, and the Workhouses*, London, 1849, p. 13.

8 R. Southey, *Sir Thomas More: or Colloquies on the Progress and Prospects of Society*, London, 1829, vol. 2, p. 319.

9 C. C. Southey (ed.) *The Life and Correspondence of the late Robert Southey*, London, 1850, vol. 6, pp. 65, 71–2.

10 A. Mozley (ed.) *Letters and Correspondence of John Henry Newman*, London, 1891, vol. 1, p. 252; Bodleian Library, MSS. Top. Oxon c. 271, Minutes of the Board of Health 1831–2, fol. 25.

11 C. C. Southey, op. cit., pp. 66–70; C. L. Brightwell, *Memorials of the Life of Mrs. Opie*, Norwich, 1854, p. 243; Aspinall, op. cit., p. 6.

12 J. Whitney, *Elizabeth Fry*, London, 1937, pp. 295–8.

13 See Lewis, op. cit.

14 The following account of the constitution and practices of the Fry Institution is drawn from the manuscript minutes of the Committee of Management, kept at the Queen's Nursing Institute, London, and from printed reports in the Bodleian Library, Oxford. Information on St John's House is drawn from printed reports in the Bodleian, the British Library and the Greater London Record Office, and from manuscript minutes and diaries kept in the Greater London Record Office (henceforth GLRO).

15 GLRO H.I./ST/SJ/A 19/1, letter of Elizabeth Frere, 1.2.1849, fol. 7.

16 Fry Minutes 1, fols 27–8, 23.7.1841. The suggestion for the change of name came from Queen Adelaide: 'I think it would prove less objectionable to many.'

17 Applications for hospital nurses figure constantly in both sisterhoods' records. On workhouse nursing, see Fry Minutes 1, fol. 49, 10.12.1841; fol. 83, 9.9.1842; Minutes 2, fol. 51b, 9.8.1844; Minutes 3, fol. 161, 16.2.1849. On the London Fever Hospital and the United Hospital, Bath, see GLRO H.I./ST/SJ/ A 35/1. In-letters 2, 3–5, 10.

18 On Mary Stanley's role in Crimean War nursing, see A. Summers, *Angels and Citizens: British Women as Military Nurses, 1854–1914*, London, 1988, ch.2.

19 M. Stanley, *Hospitals and Sisterhoods*, London, 1854, pp. 3–5.

20 Ibid., pp. 44–5.

21 Charing Cross Hospital, Minutes of the Council, fol. 45, 30.5.1865.

22 Charing Cross Hospital, Minutes of the Council, 5.4.1865; *Lancet*, 11.8.1866, p. 152; *Guardian*, 6.6.1900, p. 811.

23 British Library, Add. MSS., 43,395 f. 318, Jane Shaw Stewart to Sidney Herbert, 10.7.1861.

24 H. St G. Saunders, *The Middlesex Hospital*, London, 1949, p. 40; E. R. Frizelle and J. D. Martin, *The Leicester Royal Infirmary 1771–1971*, Leicester, 1971, pp. 139–40; S. A Plotkin 'The crisis at Guy's Hospital', *Guy's Hospital Gazette*, 1961, vol. 75.

25 Baly, op. cit., pp. 57, 61–2, 91–2, 95, 97.

26 W. Rathbone, *The Organisation of Nursing in a Large Town*, London and Liverpool, 1865, p. 34.

27 C. C. Southey, op. cit., pp. 71–2.

28 GLRO H.I./ST/SJ/A 19/2, Lady Superintendent's Reports, 6.4.1850.

29 GLRO H.I./ST/SH/A 5/1, Minutes of the House Committee, fols 156–71, May–June 1852.

30 Fry Minutes 3, fol. 183, 26.10.1849.

31 GLRO H.I./ST/SJ/A 19/1, Memorandum of Elizabeth Frere, 19.2.1849, fols 12–13.

32 Fry Register of Occupations, fols 11, 61.

33 Fry Minutes 2, fol. 62, 7.2.1845; fol. 64, 7.3.1845.

34 Fry Minutes 1, fol. 78, 16.7.1842.

35 GLRO H.I./ST/SJ/A 19/2, Lady Superintendent's Report, 17.11.1849.

36 GLRO H.I./ST/SJ/A 5/1, Minutes of the House Committee, fol. 115, 10.2.1851.

37 Fry Minutes 3, fol. 244, 14.3.1851.

38 E. J. Edwards, *A Nursing Association for the Diocese of Lichfield*,

London, 1865, p. 29.

39 See for example N. P. Blaker, *Sussex in Bygone Days*, Hove, 1919, pp. 169, 171 on Sussex County Hospital c.1864. Leicester Royal Infirmary did not employ theatre sisters until 1901 (I. C. Ellis, *Records of 19th Century Leicester*, Guernsey, 1935, p. 180); the London Hospital hardly did so before 1941 (A. E. Clark-Kennedy, *The London*, London, 1963, vol. 2, pp. 288–9).

40 S. T. Anning, *The General Infirmary at Leeds*, Leeds, 1966, vol. 2, pp. 40–1.

41 GLRO H.I./ST/SJ/C 3/1, Register of Nurses, fols 30, 46, 108.

42 Charing Cross Hospital, Minutes of the Council, fol. 258, 2.1.1867.

43 'Report on the Nursing Arrangements of the London Hospitals', *British Medical Journal*, 4 April 1874, p. 462.

44 See for example R. Richardson, *Death, Dissection and the Destitute*, London, 1987, p. 43.

45 *A Memoir of the Life of Elizabeth Fry* (edited by two of her daughters), London, 1847, vol. 2, p. 384; *Memorials of Agnes Elizabeth Jones* (by her sister), London, 1871, pp. 134–5.

46 F. B. Smith, *Florence Nightingale: Reputation and Power*, London, 1982, p. 161. Smith conveys a misleading impression that King's severed its connection with St John's House after this episode.

47 J. E. O'Neill, 'Finding a policy for the sick poor', *Victorian Studies*, 1963–4, vol. 7; G. Rivett, *The Development of the London Hospital System 1823–1982*, London, 1986, ch. 6.

9

LAY AND MEDICAL CONCEPTIONS OF MEDICAL CHARITY DURING THE NINETEENTH CENTURY

The case of the Huddersfield General Dispensary and Infirmary

Hilary Marland

Dating back to the work of Sigerist and Rosen,[1] the hospital and associated medical charities have come to be labelled as social institutions, embodying social policies and ambitions. Indeed the medical aspects of hospital development remain shadowy; 'the medicine is often ignored in histories of hospitals',[2] a result in part of the bias towards social and economic issues in nineteenth-century hospital archives. Morris Vogel, for example, has claimed that for much of the nineteenth century the American hospital was 'a largely undifferentiated welfare institution', rather than a medical environment.[3] It has been argued that the setting up of hospitals was frequently unrelated to medical needs; it cannot be 'assumed that infirmaries were created, expanded and adapted in accordance with the needs of local communities, or even that the advocates of modest medical improvements could rely on support from the wealthier classes who traditionally supported medical charities'.[4] Much early hospital development had little to do with the demands of population increase and industrialization, or associated health problems; many were founded in small county towns, not centres of rapid growth. Dispensaries to a certain extent came forward to fill this gap, but again were not necessarily set up in areas where need was the greatest, and they could not offer all the services covered by hospitals. The limits on the funding of voluntary hospitals remained a barrier to expansion throughout the nineteenth century, in-patient facilities often being particularly slow to develop (the empty hospital ward was as symbolic of this period as it is of the 1990s); the limited vision of the lay boards of management was potentially an even greater barrier.

The Huddersfield Dispensary and Infirmary was the sole charity of any significance to be set up in nineteenth-century Huddersfield – situated in the West Riding of Yorkshire – with the specific aim of providing medical assistance. Founded in 1814 in a rapidly industrializing community, the Dispensary's promoters based their claims for support on the fact that they were responding in an imaginative and efficient way to the demands of a growing labour force for health care, especially assistance in accidents and in cases of infectious disease. Later appeals for expansion to include in-patient facilities were based primarily on the need for an accident hospital. Despite these apparently clear-cut medical purposes, the functioning of the charity and admissions policies were dictated largely by social and economic criteria. Medical need and socio-economic criteria frequently overlapped – for example, there were large numbers of accidents among the labouring population – but imbalances, principally due to a large increase in demand, a result of the town's massive population growth,[5] and shortages of money, often coinciding with economic downturns and increased hardship and sickness, created problems for the charity's supporters. More desperate were the problems of those of the local population who failed to fit in with the institution's medical and socio-economic criteria: the chronically ill, the aged, the pauper.[6]

The motivations behind the establishment and support of the Huddersfield Dispensary and Infirmary, primarily then the 'lay' view of what the charity should be aiming to do, will form the starting-point of this chapter. The 'actuality' of the charity's function, as opposed to the 'intention', will also be briefly analysed. The participation of medical practitioners in voluntary hospitals was clearly one of the linchpins on which the hospitals' success depended, but on the other hand, medical practitioners benefited in a number of well-known ways from such appointments and co-operation with the lay governors.[7] The relationship between the lay governors and medical staff of the Huddersfield Infirmary developed, as in similar charities, on the basis of mutual convenience and benefit, and, more debatably, of some form of shared sympathy with the plight of the sick poor. But did medical involvement in charity go beyond career-building aspirations? Did medical practitioners share in the aims of the lay governors, or did they have a distinct set of motives in supporting medical charity? Did medical practitioners, in the same way as lay people, regard medical charities as 'social' as well as 'medical' institutions? An attempt will be made to answer these questions later; in short, to look not only at what medical practitioners got out of medical charity, but also at their own conceptions of it.

The Huddersfield and Upper Agbrigg Dispensary and Infirmary was set up in a town whose rapid nineteenth-century expansion was based almost entirely upon the textile industry. The Dispensary was founded in 1814, ostensibly to commemorate the ending of the Napoleonic Wars. More significantly, its setting up coincided with a major trade depression and associated distress resulting from the wars, which increased the strain on both poor relief and private charity. The first decade of the nineteenth century was, for Huddersfield, 'a period of great distress caused by the war, by the high prices of food, and by the introduction of machinery [in the textile industry]'.[8] In 1820 it was still being claimed that many of Huddersfield's inhabitants were destitute of food and clothing and suffering the 'severest distress'.[9] Yet at the same time, the population of the town was increasing rapidly; by over 33 per cent between 1811 and 1821, when the population passed the 13,000 mark, an expansion which was to continue well into the mid-nineteenth century.

Coincident with this – and perhaps paradoxically during such a period of depression – for reasons largely of civic pride, the citizens of Huddersfield became concerned that they were falling behind other towns in the region in the provision of medical services. By 1814 infirmaries had been set up in York (1740), Leeds (1767), Hull (1782) and Sheffield (1797); dispensaries in a larger number of Yorkshire towns, many (at least in the eyes of the Huddersfield citizenry) of less importance than Huddersfield. The build-up of civic pride in Huddersfield during the early nineteenth century was reflected in the construction of public buildings, the founding of new churches, schools and charities, and bungling attempts to improve the condition of the town, with some good results in the more conspicuous parts, with rather less determination and success in the poorer districts.[10] The first half of the nineteenth century witnessed an influx of pioneering individuals into Huddersfield, in particular cloth manufacturers, men who 'had come into the town, grown with it, moulded it, had their opportunities and perceptions enlarged by it'.[11] These individuals were largely behind town improvement and the setting up of philanthropic institutions.

By the 1830s there were thirty-two substantial wool textile mills in the parish of Huddersfield alongside numerous small-scale concerns,[12] and the town was being described as one of the four 'principal seats and emporiums of the Yorkshire woollen manufactures'.[13] The building of mills achieved even higher levels in the 1840s and 1850s. The 'energetic and persevering industry' of West Riding merchants and manufacturers, declared Edward Baines, allied to 'the highest mechanical skill, large capital and mercantile intelligence and enterprise' constituted 'the mainspring' of Britain's wealth, population and power.[14] 'We don't now live in the days of Barons, thank God,' exclaimed the Whig politician Brougham in the Leeds Cloth Hall Yard in 1830, 'we live in the days of Leeds, of Bradford, of Halifax and of Huddersfield.'[15] The ethics of self-advancement, enterprise and industry – 'pulling oneself up by the bootstraps' – were nowhere stronger than in Huddersfield. It was, despite the recent disruption of the wars and trade depression, into this atmosphere of growth, optimism, civic improvement and dynamism that the Huddersfield Dispensary was born in 1814.

Huddersfield, perhaps best described as a 'frontier' town during this period, had a limited basis from which to start a major charitable enterprise – no experience and no build-up of philanthropic expertise, and also no preconceptions concerning the form the charity should take. From the start, the Dispensary came to be dominated by the causes and products of Huddersfield's early nineteenth-century expansion. The vast majority of officers and committee members were local merchants and manufacturers. Out of the first committee of eighteen members, all but two were involved in the textile industry. Especially active were J. M. Ridgway (wool-stapler), Henry Stables (woollen merchant and manufacturer), two members of the Battye family (cloth manufacturers) and John Fisher (silk spinner). The committee was perhaps even more notable for its omissions: no clergymen served on the committee, no professionals – its first treasurers were, unusually, not bankers nor legal practitioners, but woollen merchants and manufacturers, Messrs Brook and Sons – and no members of the local gentry.[16]

The reasoning behind the establishment and ongoing support of the Huddersfield Dispensary, and later its extension into an

Infirmary, cannot be reduced to a monocausal explanation. Pragmatic and economic considerations were the most important of the wide spectrum of motivations behind the founding of the charity, which included social, economic, political, religious and humanitarian feelings as well as a desire, in the face of the threats and periodic actuality of popular uprisings, to ameliorate the conditions of the poor. The main expedient was to provide a cheap and efficient form of medical relief for cases among the sick poor, caused particularly by accidents, suffered for the most part by the employees of local manufacturers, and by infectious diseases, which threatened to invade the homes of the wealthier classes, and become a burden on ratepayers and employers. In common with most eighteenth- and nineteenth-century medical charities, admission policies were largely dictated by social, not medical, criteria, with emphasis being placed on treating the 'deserving poor' and 'proper objects', translatable as 'those with a role to play in the local economy'. This made much sense to the charity's supporters, if not to the sick poor who fell outside these boundaries. Emphasis was placed on restoring the workman to his calling, a factor of special importance in an area 'whose local Prosperity is so intimately interwoven with the Maintenance of the Health and Strength of the laborious Poor'.[17] While the geographical scope of the charity was wide and fairly unrestricted, subscribers were constantly being warned about the pitfalls – social and even moral, but chiefly financial – of admitting those not entitled to its benefits. Yet although socio-economic factors played a crucial role in determining who would and who would not be admitted, medical criteria were also strictly defined, particularly with reference to in-patient admissions – acute, surgical and accident cases had priority over chronic and medical conditions; 'incurables', pregnant women, illnesses associated with old age, venereal diseases and lunacy were totally unacceptable in the in-patients department, and such cases were accepted only with reluctance as out-patients.[18]

While the thread tying together the motives of the Dispensary's supporters is possible to detect from the start, the annual reports reveal a curious mixture of altruism, Christian benevolence, tempered paternalism and pure pragmatism. Policy-making was very much dominated by one group, the merchants and manufacturers, who had few rivals in the charitable field and few charities competing for support, yet the net had to be thrown wide in attracting funding. The first annual report of the Dispensary stated that within ten months 'twelve hundred objects' had been relieved:

> The Importance of the industrious Poor, to a mercantile
> District like this, would of itself entitle them to the special
> Guardianship of their more opulent Neighbours, if the still
> more holy, and more commanding Voice of Charity did not
> furnish a nobler Incentive.[19]

The institution could not fulfil the ambitions of its supporters
and needs of the district for long, and a purpose-built Infirmary
was established in connection with the Dispensary in 1831, only
seventeen years after the founding of the Dispensary. In 1823 the
committee, in pressing for an infirmary, appealed both to notions
of pragmatism and the more 'old-fashioned' beliefs concerning the
philanthropic duties of the wealthy, drawing

> the Attention of the Governors to the Expediency of providing
> a Fund for the Erection of Wards, for the Reception of a limited
> Number of In-Patients; more especially for those frequent
> Accidents arising from the extensive Use of Machinery. . . .
> In a District distinguished for its pious Munificence, there will
> not be wanting Individuals, blessed with the Will as well as
> with the Means, to atchieve [sic] this Work of Philanthropy;
> and who, as Stewards of Heaven's Bounty, deem it their best
> Gain to dedicate their Wealth to the Service of Charity, and
> reap its Fruits in due Season, in that better Country, where
> Talents thus laid out will bear Interest to all Eternity.[20]

The returns on an investment in medical charity were claimed to be
superior to those offered by other forms of philanthropy. The jargon
of commerce was much utilized in appeals for support, with reference
being made to 'maximum utility' and 'value for money' in return for
a modest investment in the 'Joint-Stock bank of Charity'.[21] Medical
charity prevented pauperization, and was

> not subject to the abuses and imposition that too often attach
> to the relief of mere destitution. It husbands the resources
> of society when viewed in reference to the mitigation of
> suffering, the speedy return of the workman to his labour,
> and the probable diminution of the loss of life.[22]

Any number of objections can be raised concerning an over-reliance
on annual reports or fund-raising propaganda as statements of
intention or of policy. Such material exaggerated the success of the

charity, being largely intended to encourage support. Self-flattery and flattery of supporters took precedence. However, there are a number of other ways of assessing the policies of medical charities, the aims of their supporters, and their success in fulfilling these aims. If we look first in more detail at the nature of support, at those individuals and groups playing a leading role in managing or funding the charity, and at the annual subscribers who supplied the bread and butter support upon which the institution depended, we find that both groups were heavily concentrated in commerce, especially the textile industry. Prominent supporters of the Huddersfield Infirmary included Sir Joseph Armitage, a local woollen mill owner and deputy-lieutenant for the West Riding, who lent his name to the charity by accepting the posts of vice-president and subsequently president in 1836. Armitage had been especially active in the campaign to establish the Infirmary. Others, such as Charles Brook, a cotton thread and silk manufacturer, confined their contributions to supplying money, in his case a massive £30,000 to build a convalescent home in connection with the Infirmary, while playing a limited role in management and policy direction. Numerous individuals participated at a lower level of managerial and financial involvement, as benefactors, fund-raisers and committee members; the textile interest was also well-represented at this level. All such individuals, whatever other motives they might have had for involvement, had a vested interest in supplying efficient medical aid for their employees.

An occupational analysis of subscribers to the Huddersfield Dispensary and Infirmary reveals, not surprisingly, that, in addition to the leadership of the charity, the hard core of support came from commercial groups, primarily those involved in the manufacturing or marketing of textiles. To take just one year, in 1865–6 the number of merchants and manufacturers subscribing to the charity was 272 (53.2 per cent of all subscribers). Those occupied within the textile industry made up over 80 per cent of subscribing merchants and manufacturers. The next largest group of supporters were tradesmen, who made up 24.3 per cent of subscribers. Subscribers were spread thinly over other occupational groupings, including service groups (5.3 per cent), 'gentlemen' (4.1 per cent), clergymen and ministers (2.9 per cent) and farmers (0.2 per cent).[23]

The concentration on accident and disease cases was reflected not only in declared admissions policies, but also in actual admissions, albeit to a lesser extent. Accidents, the only category which could be admitted directly without a subscriber's recommendation, represented a large proportion of all cases treated by the charity, this applying especially to in-patient admissions. Indeed, initially the in-patients department came to cater almost exclusively for 'accidents and cases of immediate exigence'. In the Infirmary's first year of operation, 1831–2, admissions included an

> unusual number of accidents so serious as to admit of no delay
> . . . among its first fruits, in the short space since the wards were opened, there have been eighteen cases of fracture, many of a serious description, admitted, and no less than 12 amputations besides various other important operations performed, and a considerable number of accidents relieved within the Infirmary.
> . . . And who that has observed the rapid rate of increase of our population, the growing use of machinery, and its necessary results, the increase of accidents, that will not feel on this ground that the Charity is entitled to his best support.[24]

In 1846–7 379 accident cases were admitted, an average of more than one case a day.[25] In 1864 the committee drew the attention of the subscribers to the 'excessive number' of cases of scalds, fractures and severe accidents.[26] Timothy Holmes, who visited the Infirmary in the same year, confirmed that accident cases made up the majority of in-patient admissions.[27]

In 1873–4 accident cases still made up 34 per cent of in-patient admissions. Half of the fifty-five operations performed in this year were amputations; eighty-five cases of fracture and dislocation were also admitted as in-patients, and there were sixty-three wounds, contusions and sprains.[28] By the year 1908–9, despite a gradual reduction in accident cases, over two thousand people with major injuries were being admitted as in-patients and casualties.[29] Once the policy of admitting a high proportion of accident cases was taken up, it became self-perpetuating; accident cases quickly filled up the available beds,[30] and were tedious to treat.

Several factors conspired, however, against the charity functioning solely, or even chiefly, as an accident hospital, and against the strict implementation of other medical and socio-economic admissions policies. The cost of treating accident cases was prohibitive; the returns, in terms of the high mortality rates associated with accidents, unacceptable. The admission of other categories of case, especially as out-patients, helped balance the figures. As the only major medical charity in Huddersfield and the surrounding area, the institution was forced to function to some extent as a general hospital. This applied especially to the Dispensary department, which came to cater for a wide range of medical and surgical cases as out- or home-patients. The town had no fever hospital, and the Dispensary treated large numbers of infectious disease cases, especially in epidemic years.

In effect, the charity developed as two parallel institutions, the Dispensary department being more responsive to local health problems, treating a wide range of complaints, and significantly larger numbers than the Infirmary. In 1860–1, for example, 3,787 out-patients were admitted and 176 in-patients; the ratio of in- to out-patients was 1:22, and this was not untypical.[31] The Infirmary department, meanwhile, functioned to some extent as the 'symbolic' expression of medical charity, for much of the century, having little impact on the health of the community. In 1861 the annual report indicated that almost 11 per cent of the inhabitants of Huddersfield township had received Dispensary treatment in the past year, compared with the 0.5 per cent admitted as in-patients.[32]

Not only the needs of the local populace, but also the demands of the hospital's medical staff for a wider range of services, led to their expansion. As medical science advanced, more opportunities became available for treating and curing. Slowly the wide scope of out-patient care began to be matched by in-patient provision. By the end of the century, cases of rheumatism, bronchitis, phthisis, heart disease, cancer and a variety of 'female disorders' were being admitted as in-patients. Emphasis was still on surgical and acute cases, but the range of complaints dealt with expanded annually.

A final way in which admission policies were reflected was in the class of patients admitted. As with most dispensaries and infirmaries of this period, patient records for the Huddersfield Infirmary are virtually non-existent, either in the form of details of admissions and treatment, or, aside from isolated complaints procedures, describing the patients' experiences of medical charity. One of the few pieces of information we have on the social and occupational class of patients admitted to the Huddersfield Infirmary, consists of the lists of in-patients recorded in the census enumerators' books for the years 1841 to 1881 (Table 1).[33] The enumerators' books provide a snapshot of patient admissions, the listings recording, for example, 15 per cent of the total admissions in the year 1860–1, 10 per cent of admissions in 1880–1. Textile workers accounted for a high proportion of admissions in each year; 57 per cent in 1841, 47 per cent in 1861, but perhaps less than we might expect from the charity's propaganda.[34] Other patients were for the most part gainfully employed in the local economy, namely miscellaneous labourers and artisans, while a small number were servants. Women and children with no recorded occupation were also admitted, but very few unemployed men. None of the patients in the sample was recorded as a pauper, the governors of the Infirmary actively discouraging this class of admission.[35]

Table 1 Occupations of Huddersfield Infirmary in-patients on census day, 1841–81

Occupations	1841		1851		1861		1871		1881	
Textile workers	17	(57%)	11	(39%)	25	(47%)	2	(22%)	20	(27%)
Other factory workers	2		0		1		0		3	
General labourers	0		1		2		2		3	
Miners/ quarrymen	0		0		1		0		4	
Agricultural labourers	2		0		3		0		1	
Watermen	3		0		0		0		1	
Building trades	2		3		3		0		1	
Shoemakers	0		1		1		2		0	
Tailors/ seamstresses	0		1		3		0		0	
Hawkers	1		1		2		0		2	
Servants	1		3		5		0		7	
Males (no occupation)	0		0		1		0		3	
Females (no occupation)	0		2		3		2		12	
Children (no occupation)	2		5		3		1		16	
Total	30		28		53		9		73	

Source: Census enumerators' books, Huddersfield township, 1841–81

Also significant was the age at which patients were admitted, the committee stressing that large numbers of children and adults were cured 'who have not passed the meridian of Life'.[36] A breakdown of in-patients according to age for the year 1838–9 shows how much emphasis was placed on admitting those involved in the local economy. The majority were male (73 per cent) and young. While only 8 per cent were less than 10 years old, over 24 per cent of admissions were aged between 10 and 20, 27 per cent between 20 and 30. Some 15 per cent were aged between 30 and 40, 11 per cent each were aged 40 to 50 and 50 to 60. Only 4 per cent were over 60.[37]

The vital importance of hospital posts to the careers of aspiring medical men has been very much stressed in hospital histories and studies of the medical profession;[38] perhaps even over-stressed at the expense of a neglect of other appointments and paths to a successful career.[39] There is no doubt that medical practitioners were very much helped on their way by an honorary hospital post, in terms of practice-building opportunities, social prestige, clinical experience, the ability to take on pupils, and to develop a consulting practice. One suspects, however, that what was true for London and other major cities cannot necessarily be applied to the provincial situation, at least in terms of the scale of the benefits.

In Huddersfield medical practitioners would have to be already in something of an elite position in the local medical and social hierarchy before they acquired an honorary post.[40] The interplay between social contacts, voluntary society and other community activities, and appointment to hospital posts was of great significance. Being a 'local man' was perhaps the factor of most importance.[41] There was a residency requirement of at least one year before an individual could be appointed honorary medical officer to the Huddersfield Infirmary, and only occasionally was this rule relaxed, as in the case of the appointment of Dr John Taylor, ex-professor of clinical medicine and physician to University College Hospital, London, who was elected honorary physician in 1846. An honorary appointee would preferably be Huddersfield born and raised, at best a member of a medical dynasty, but, if not, of a sound family background. Many, especially after the mid-nineteenth century, had familial connections with the woollen trade, the sons of manufacturers often taking up one of the learned professions. The new commercial classes not only created the largest part of the demand for medical care, but also came forward to fill it. A large proportion of honorary appointees, as part of the process of familiarization, would have already served a term as house surgeon to the institution.

In 1884 Mr Norman Porritt, son of Jabez William Porritt of Clare Hill, Huddersfield, a 'pioneer of the wool trade', offered his services as honorary surgeon to the Infirmary, 'soliciting, as a native of Huddersfield, your support and votes'.[42] Nephew of Councillor Richard Porritt, grandson of the late Mr James Astin, a respected

Huddersfield surgeon, Norman Porritt had been educated at the Huddersfield Collegiate School and Leeds University, and had served as senior assistant house surgeon to the Leeds Infirmary.[43] After returning to Huddersfield, he was appointed senior house surgeon to the Huddersfield Infirmary (out of twenty-four applicants).[44] Resigning his house surgeoncy after a three-year term, Porritt took up residence on the New North Road, close to the Infirmary. With such impeccable qualifications, he could not fail to be successful.[45] He joined the seven other honorary staff, all of whom were resident in Huddersfield when appointed; four of these men were natives of Yorkshire, and three, like Porritt, had been born in Huddersfield.[46] Porritt retained his honorary post until 1911, a period of twenty-seven years. He was appointed chairman of the Huddersfield division of the BMA, and president of the Huddersfield Medical Society. Porritt's obituary in the *Huddersfield Examiner* in March, 1940 described him glowingly as 'one of the most popular practitioners Huddersfield ever had'.[47]

Although other qualities were important – high professional status in the form of a string of impressive and 'gentlemanly' qualifications, especially university degrees, and college and medical society attachments[48] – local connections do not seem to have decreased in significance as the century progressed. Many posts were not even advertised in the major medical journals, it being thought adequate to solicit applications through the local press. In 1905 all twelve candidates for the three posts of honorary physician, ophthalmic and aural surgeon, and honorary general surgeon resided in Huddersfield. Six were neighbours, residing in New North Road, the 'Harley Street' of Huddersfield, where the Infirmary was also sited.[49]

An obituary which appeared in the *Lancet* in 1910, marking the death of Thomas Kilner Clarke, MD, late honorary surgeon to the Huddersfield Infirmary, stressed the importance of local connections and family ties. Born in Huddersfield in 1843, the notice declared, 'Dr. Clarke was *bred up* to join the medical profession' (my emphasis).[50] His father, William James Clarke, had one of the leading practices in the town, to which Thomas succeeded at the age of 28, and which he subsequently extended. 'Dr. Clarke came to his work well equipped', as a Cambridge graduate and a Guy's man, completing his studies in Paris, and obtaining various hospital posts in London before 'he returned to Huddersfield, where his abilities were soon recognized and he was chosen for the first vacancy on the infirmary staff. He held the appointment of surgeon to the infirmary till his death.'[51]

Honorary posts implied the sacrifice of time, medical practitioners not only giving medical assistance gratis, but also participating in the management of the Infirmary, serving as *ex-officio* board members, and involving themselves at all levels from participation in sub-committees and fund-raising to ordering beds, drugs and leeches, and inspecting drains! Most medical officers retained their positions for a great many years; Dr William Scott for forty years, Dr William Turnbull for sixty, George Robinson for fifty-six years, his son William for forty. By so doing, they made it difficult for new openings to be created for young medical practitioners, especially 'outsiders'.

While testimonials to their hard work abound, in general medical practitioners have left few records describing their views on medical charity, aside from complaints concerning the abuses of hospitals, particularly within the out-patients departments, and the consequent loss of paying patients. Those actively involved in medical charities were remarkably reticent concerning their motives for devoting so much time and energy to such work, without remuneration, often for lengthy periods of time. For the Huddersfield case, where medical practitioners have left details explaining the importance of medical charity as they saw it, their views bore close resemblance to the statements of the lay supporters, and were dominated by social rather than medical imperatives.

In 1825 when Dr Turnbull, physician to the Dispensary, drew up an appeal on behalf of the intended hospital at Huddersfield, he stressed the necessity of isolating infectious disease cases, and the role of medical charities in stepping in to prevent pauperism and dependence upon the rates, and in offsetting poor living and working conditions. Little mention was made by Turnbull or others of strictly medical imperatives, the need to provide a sanitary environment, nursing attendance or to monitor patients, or even details of the kind of cases which they believed would benefit from hospitalization.[52] Similarly at the ceremonies marking the laying of the foundation stone of the Infirmary in 1829 and the opening of the new building in 1831, the statements of the medical practitioners present were barely distinguishable from those of the lay supporters. In 1829 Mr Favell, surgeon to the Leeds Infirmary, emphasized the necessity of 'using great discrimination in the admission of patients'. Dr Turnbull reminded the gathering of the need to step up charitable efforts in times of distress.[53] Two years later, at the opening ceremony, Turnbull also warned of the problems involved in running such a charity.

> Difficulties we must expect, but if we are prudent in the management ... if we do not attempt too much ... do not indulge in acts of overexertion ... we shall maintain our situation, and realize our expectations. ... Economy and friends will long be necessary.

Turnbull held very much to traditional notions of charity: 'The rich require the services of the poor, and the poor the patronage and support of the rich'.[54] Dr Walker spoke of 'the ties of harmony and good-will' created through involvement in medical charity;[55] infirmaries 'present a common ground upon which we can all meet'. He went on to describe infirmaries as

> monuments of the benevolence of past ages, equally an honour to the rich, and a blessing to the poor. And can you harbour a doubt that the same will be the case with our own institution, supported by a vast population in a town too whose commerce is co-extensive with the limits of the habitable globe, and whose hand was never closed against the wants of the poor![56]

It is impossible to assess how much such statements were truly reflective of the feelings of the profession concerning medical charity. Or were they bowing to necessity? It is important to remember, however, that these individuals already had appointments which they were not likely to lose. The pressure on them to conform may have been less than we would imagine.

Some sections of the medical profession opted out of or were unable to gain entry to the Infirmary.[57] Inability to obtain an appointment generally led to an unwillingness to support the institution in other ways. While the honorary medical officers frequently gave financial support, such as the 'handsome donation' of £50 paid by Dr Turnbull in 1836,[58] few non-appointees subscribed or donated to the charity. Five medical practitioners subscribed to the institution in the year 1830–1 (3.4 per cent of subscribers), thirteen in 1865–6 (but only 2.5 per cent of subscribers).[59] Just three medical practitioners were recorded as having made donations to the special fund for the building of the Huddersfield Infirmary: Dr Walker, physician to the charity and a prominent campaigner for its extension, Dr James Bradley, ex-honorary physician, and Dr Caleb

Crowther, physician to the Dispensary in nearby Wakefield and an important local philanthropist.[60]

Others were apparently opposed in principle to the idea of medical charity. One such individual was Samuel Knaggs, a Huddersfield general practitioner, and strong advocate of self-help dispensaries and insurance societies. At the AGM of the Huddersfield Infirmary in 1859, Knaggs proposed that the governors should investigate the possibilities of self-help medical provision for the poor of the town as an alternative to medical charity.[61] In the same year he wrote to the *Medical Times and Gazette* suggesting the setting up of insurance societies for the poor and working classes, to which every qualified regular doctor could be attached.[62] Knaggs's suggestion to the Infirmary governors was rejected out of hand, and Knaggs appears to have overcome any scruples he may have had concerning medical charity when he was appointed to the post of honorary surgeon a few years later, in 1863.[63] Knaggs's connections with the Infirmary were long-standing. He had married into a local textile dynasty, and his father-in-law, John Battye, had been the charity's first honorary secretary, his brother-in-law, T. H. Battye, for many years an active board member.[64] Knaggs became an archetypal honorary medical officer, a member of the monthly and building committees. He was president of the Yorkshire Branch of the BMA, active in the Huddersfield Medical Society and local voluntary societies, publishing on a wide variety of medical subjects directed at both the general and medical public, and founding a dynasty of honorary infirmary surgeons. Two of his three sons followed him into practice; one, Dr Lawford Knaggs, in Leeds, and the other, Dr Francis Henry Knaggs, in Huddersfield. Francis was appointed ophthalmic and aural surgeon to the Infirmary in 1905, and built up a flourishing private practice. When Samuel Knaggs died in 1911, the 'oldest surgeon in Huddersfield' and honorary surgeon to the Infirmary for thirty-five years, he left an estate and personal property valued at well over £8,000, perhaps the surest sign of professional success.[65]

In many ways, it is not surprising that medical practitioners shared the lay conception of medical charity. They were, after all, for the most part members of the same class as the lay governors, with overlapping ideas on society and philanthropy. Within the community, alliances were formed with others of the middle class through political and religious affiliations, and civic and voluntary society activities.[66] Those medical practitioners most active in these fields were likely to be honorary appointees. Medical practitioners were influenced strongly by the local environment, and shared in the business interests of the community, many having direct family links through descent or marriage with local manufacturers. Norman Porritt's commercial background, and Samuel Knaggs's links through marriage to the textile interest, have already been referred to. Medical men were also in the business of making money, and the success of their practices was tied up with the success of the local economy, and the fortunes of their clientele. They shared in the gospels of improvement and gain, powerful influences in towns such as Huddersfield; Samuel Smiles, the high priest of self-help, had himself been a Yorkshire medical practitioner. Medical practitioners too, early in the century, had for the most part been 'frontier' men, carving out their practices as newcomers to the town. The obituary of Thomas Kilner Clarke, mentioned above, praised him for his great industry and his accumulation of a large number of medical posts in addition to a busy practice, and for being 'a shrewd man of business – he was a Yorkshireman'![67]

Local doctors shared to some extent in the cynicism and modest paternalism which was associated with medical charity in communities such as Huddersfield. Many members of the medical profession were associated with the Whig interest, which dominated party politics in Huddersfield for much of the century, linking themselves by implication to the anti-Factory Act lobby (and to support for the Anatomy Act).[68] Dr John Kenworthy Walker, physician to the Infirmary from 1814 to 1846, was one of the few medical practitioners to come out in outspoken criticism of the factory system. He was a supporter of the Factory Movement and an ally of Richard Oastler, then active in Huddersfield. In 1831 Dr Walker condemned those who treated man as 'a manufacturing animal', and urged masters to act as the 'moral guardians of this great family', describing the 'competitive system' as 'a state of Commercial cannibalism, or suicidal system of commerce!'[69] Despite Walker's fierce denunciations of the factory system, by working for medical charity and alongside local manufacturers, he helped perpetuate it. Medical charity, after all, relieved manufacturers from the obligation of making the work-place safe and healthy, and from providing some form of direct medical cover for their employees. In the same year as he made the above statements, Walker was busy campaigning for the establishment of the Infirmary to treat accident cases, victims of the factory system.

Medical practitioners were forced to tread a fine line in their involvement in medical charity; there was potentially a conflict of interest. On the one hand, many social and professional advantages were obtained through Infirmary posts. On the other, medical practitioners wished to limit the scope of the charity, and especially to minimize the risk of losing paying patients. They therefore directly shared in many of the concerns of the lay committee, being anxious to refuse admission to certain social or medical categories, such as Poor Law patients, chronic cases and incurables, and certainly those wealthy enough to pay for private treatment. The question of the abuse of the charity came regularly to the fore, as in 1884 when the issue arose following the Infirmary board's receipt of a memorial from the honorary medical officers and other local medical practitioners, which stated that a large number of out-patients had been recommended who were well able to pay for medical assistance. The same memorial opposed the proposal of the Infirmary board to increase the number of honorary medical staff;

> such action is no remedy for the evil complained of, but must of necessity aggravate it, because any such increase in the number of the Staff will be looked upon by the public as a further invitation to the well-to-do to avail themselves of the proffered and gratuitous Medical advice.[70]

The *Lancet* offered its support to the complainants: 'It is well known that persons who are fully able to pay the ordinary fee for professional advice are in the habit of procuring gratuitous medical relief at the infirmary'.[71] Steps were taken by the Infirmary board to check up on patients, a standard scale being introduced and the Charity Organization Society being called in to assist, but the lay board believed that their medical officers exaggerated the extent of the abuses. At the same time, the board proceeded with the appointment of an additional surgeon, thus, in the eyes of the honorary medical officers, further extending the scope of the charity and the scope of its abusers, particularly in the out-patients department, and thus 'slighting and ignoring the opinion and wishes of the professional staff'.[72] In later years, the fear of the honorary medical officers concerning the loss of paying patients again manifested itself, in the form of fierce opposition to the introduction of the 1911 National Insurance Act.

Did the position of medical appointees to the Huddersfield Infirmary change over time, either in terms of power, or a divergence from the views and policies of the lay governors? By the late

nineteenth century, medical practitioners had achieved more professional authority on a local, as well as national, basis, by means of
improved levels of education and qualification, and their tightly
organized medical society and regional professional activities. Many
honorary medical officers had already held house surgeoncies
or more prestigious hospital appointments, often in London or
Scotland, but increasingly in Leeds, following training at the Leeds
Medical School, before their move or return to Huddersfield.
But perhaps of more importance, they had, over the decades,
consolidated their position in civic life and elite society.[73]

By the late nineteenth century medical families had made their
impact, and many of those in practice in the town were second or
third generation, truly 'local' men. They were involved in more civic
activities in larger numbers, and were highly integrated. Involvement
in medical charity was one of the avenues to increased acceptability,
and offered medical practitioners an opportunity to work together
with members of the local hierarchy and business community, the
two being largely indistinguishable in Huddersfield. It could be
argued that the profession's 'marginality'[74] was in part broken down
by the involvement of doctors in medical charity, and their apparent
willingness to co-operate with the lay officers in policy and aims.

At an internal level, by late in the century, the medical staff had
recognizably more say at committee meetings and in policy-making.
The power of the honorary medical officers increased in subtle ways;
they served in larger numbers on the board, which became more
likely to act upon their recommendations, they served on more
sub-committees, including building and rule-devising committees,
and occasionally they were permitted to bring their private patients
to the Infirmary for treatment. Their increased impact on decision-
making meant that they also had more say in the allocation of funds.
In 1881, for example, the honorary medical staff advised the board
to erect a sanatorium for isolation cases, which was carried out
at the cost of almost £250. Although the board felt the expense
to be considerable, they were also convinced that 'the building
is absolutely necessary for the welfare of the patients treated in
the institution'.[75] Another landmark was reached in 1871 with the
proposal to name a new ward the 'Turnbull Ward', 'out of respect
to Dr. Turnbull and his prominent services'.[76] William Turnbull had
served the charity as honorary physician from 1816, and continued
in his post till within a few weeks of his death in 1876. He was also
honoured with a board-room portrait in 1863, a banquet to celebrate

the fiftieth year of his connection with the Infirmary in 1867, a gift of silver plate on his formal resignation, and a dedication in the form of a plaque on the newly erected medicated baths in 1876.[77]

The more important position of medical practitioners in the Infirmary machine was confirmed by the setting up of a medical committee towards the end of the century (whose earliest records have alas not survived). The influence of medical practitioners peaked with the appointment in 1914 of Dr F. W. Robinson as president of the Infirmary, the first medical practitioner to be selected for this post. On the other hand, lay people still largely retained control over admissions, and the honorary medical officers were permitted to retain only small numbers of patients on the books at a time. Worse still, the selection of honorary medical officers, the house surgeon, and nursing staff remained chiefly in the hands of the infirmary board and governors. Though many barriers between the medical profession and the lay governors had been broken down, others remained in force. Financial and executive power remained firmly in lay hands.

The unity of the honorary medical officers with the lay policy-makers reflected a degree of agreement concerning the purposes of medical charity; medical practitioners to some extent also saw voluntary dispensaries and infirmaries as social institutions, sorting offices which would leave paying patients for their private practices. How much this collusion was due to the social and professional needs felt by medical practitioners for honorary posts, or how much this was based on genuine agreement, is hard to estimate. In the end, it is as difficult to be definite about the policy statements of medical practitioners as of lay people, but perhaps it is wrong to assume that medical practitioners' involvement was based solely on professional advantage. Huddersfield, its economy being based heavily on textiles, and the policy-making machinery and financial support of the charity being so much based on textile money, is hardly a typical case. But such an example perhaps highlights the potential of examining medical charity in a local context, showing that the interests of medical groups were closely connected with the local economy and society, medical practitioners' notions of medical charity interweaving with those of lay groups.

Acknowledgements

The author would like to thank the staff of the Kirklees District

Archives and Local Studies Department, and of the West Yorkshire County Record Office.

NOTES

1 See for example H. Sigerist, 'An outline of the development of the hospital', *Bulletin of the History of Medicine*, 1936, vol. 4; G. Rosen, 'The hospital: historical sociology of a community institution', in Rosen, *From Medical Police to Social Medicine: Essays on the History of Health Care*, New York, 1974.

2 L. Granshaw, *St Mark's Hospital, London: A Social History of a Specialist Hospital*, Oxford, 1985, p. xv.

3 M. J. Vogel, 'The transformation of the American hospital, 1850–1920', in S. Reverby and D. Rosner (eds) *Health Care in America: Essays in Social History*, Philadelphia, 1979, p. 105. See also Vogel's monograph *The Invention of the Modern Hospital*, Chicago and London, 1980.

4 C. Webster, 'The crisis of the hospitals during the industrial revolution', in E. Forbes (ed.) *Human Implications of Scientific Advance*, Edinburgh, 1978, p. 214.

5 From 7,268 in 1801, to 25,068 in 1841, 38,654 in 1871, and 44,921 by 1901 (Huddersfield township); W. Page, *The Victoria History of the County of York*, vol. 3, London, 1913, p. 525.

6 For an overview of medical provisions in nineteenth-century Huddersfield, see H. Marland, *Medicine and Society in Wakefield and Huddersfield 1780–1870*, Cambridge, 1987.

7 Outlined, for example, in J. Woodward, *To Do the Sick No Harm: A Study of the British Voluntary Hospital System to 1875*, London, 1974, ch. 4, and M. J. Peterson, *The Medical Profession in Mid-Victorian London*, Berkeley, Calif., 1978, ch. 4.

8 T. Baines, *Yorkshire, Past and Present . . .*, London, 1871–7, vol. 2, p. 430.

9 *Wakefield and Halifax Journal*, 14 January 1820.

10 The Minutes of Proceedings on a Preliminary Inquiry on the Huddersfield Improvement Bill, Held February, 1848, MS, Kirklees District Archives (KHT9/1), contain numerous examples of poor housing and sanitary conditions.

11 C. Binfield, 'Asquith: the formation of a Prime Minister', *The Journal: United Reformed Church History Society*, 1981, vol. 2, no. 7, p. 219.

12 D. T. Jenkins, *The West Riding Wool Textile Industry 1770–1835*, Edington, Wiltshire, 1975, p. 24.

13 W. White, *History, Gazetteer, and Directory, of the West Riding of Yorkshire*, Sheffield, 1837, p. 360.

14 A. Briggs, *Victorian Cities*, Harmondsworth, 1968, p. 143.

15 Ibid.

16 *Annual Report of the Huddersfield Dispensary, 1814–15*, Annual Reports located at the West Yorkshire County Record Office (C500/1/33–44).

17 Ibid.

18 *Rules and Regulations of the Huddersfield and Upper Agbrigg Infirmary, 1834*, pp. 16–18, Kirklees Central Library, Local History (B. 362).
19 *Annual Report of the Huddersfield Dispensary , 1814–15.*
20 Ibid., *1822–3.*
21 *Annual Report of the Huddersfield Dispensary and Infirmary*, 1838–9.
22 Ibid., *1862–3.*
23 Ibid., *1865–6*; W. White, *Directory of Leeds, Bradford, Huddersfield, Halifax, Wakefield, Dewsbury*, Sheffield, 1866. For more details of annual subscribers, see Marland, op. cit., pp. 114–22.
24 *Annual Report of the Huddersfield Dispensary and Infirmary, 1831–2.*
25 Ibid., *1846–7.*
26 Ibid., *1863–4.*
27 PP, *Sixth Report of the Medical Officer of the Privy Council*, 1864 XXVIII I (3416), App. 15, pp. 649–50.
28 *Annual Report of the Huddersfield Dispensary and Infirmary, 1873–4.*
29 Ibid., *1908–9.*
30 Twenty beds in 1832, thirty-five in 1839, and eighty-five in 1885.
31 *Annual Report of the Huddersfield Dispensary and Infirmary, 1860–1.* Between 1831, and the addition of in-patient wards, and 1871 the ratio of in- to out-patients averaged out at 1:15. Marland, op. cit., p. 101.
32 Ibid., p. 105. For problems with patients' statistics, see ibid., pp. 103–6, 397–9, and W. Turnbull, 'Hospital Expenditure', *British Medical Journal*, 1860, pp. 656–7.
33 Census enumerators' books, Huddersfield township, 1841–81.
34 The 1871 census listed over 50 per cent of the inhabitants of Huddersfield as textile workers. Yet, in 1871 only 22 per cent of the patients listed as being resident in the hospital on census night were employed in textiles. Of course, the sample may not be representative, but the anomaly is interesting. The census data were taken from Baines, op. cit., p. 438.
35 For relations between the Infirmary governors and Poor Law officials, see Marland, op. cit., esp. pp. 63, 85–6, 92–3.
36 *Annual Report of the Huddersfield Dispensary, 1815–16.*
37 The division among out-patients was very different. Women made up over 56 per cent of out-patient admissions, and patients were distributed more evenly across the age categories. For example only 15 per cent of out-patients were aged between 20 and 30, a percentage equalled by those in the 40–50 age category, and 9 per cent of out-patients were aged over 60, twice the percentage for in-patients. *Annual Report of the Huddersfield Dispensary and Infirmary, 1838–9.*
38 See, in particular, I. Waddington, 'General practitioners and consultants in early nineteenth-century England: the sociology of an intra-professional conflict', in J. Woodward and D. Richards (eds) *Health Care and Popular Medicine in Nineteenth Century England: Essays in the Social History of Medicine*, London, 1977, esp. pp. 170–3, and Waddington, *The Medical Profession in the Industrial Revolution*, Dublin, 1984, pp. 29–49.
39 For the range of appointments in nineteenth-century Huddersfield, see Marland, op. cit., pp. 274–80.

40 Comparable with the need Peterson singled out to be an 'old boy', an ex-student, to obtain appointment to senior London hospital posts. Peterson, op. cit., pp. 141–3.

41 For the importance of locality on a regional basis, see H. Marland and P. Swan, 'Medical practice in the West Riding during the mid-nineteenth century', in D. Foster and P. Swan (eds) *Essays in Regional and Local History*, Hull, 1991 (an extension of Marland and Swan, 'West Riding medical practice from nineteenth-century census data: a view of the region and selected towns', *Bulletin of the Society for the Social History of Medicine*, 1987, no. 41) and Swan, 'Medical provision in the West Riding in 1851 and 1871' (unpublished Ph.D thesis, Humberside College of Higher Education, Hull, 1988).

42 *Testimonials in Favour of Mr. Norman Porritt, For the Office of Honorary Surgeon to the Huddersfield Infirmary*, Kirklees Central Library, Local History (Local Pamphlets 22, A080).

43 *Yorkshire Who's Who: The County Series of Who's Who in the United Kingdom, 1912*, London, 1912, p. 316.

44 Minute Book of the Huddersfield Dispensary and Infirmary, vol. 3, Monthly Board, 13 September 1880. Minute Books located at the West Yorkshire County Record Office (C500/1/1–6).

45 Ibid., Special General Meeting, 26 November 1884.

46 *Annual Report of the Huddersfield Dispensary and Infirmary, 1884–5*; Census enumerators' books, Huddersfield township, 1881.

47 *Huddersfield Examiner*, 6 March 1940.

48 For the close ties between the honorary Infirmary officers and local medical societies, see H. Marland, 'Early nineteenth-century medical society activity: the Huddersfield case', *Journal of Regional and Local Studies*, 1985, vol. 6.

49 Printed notice, dated 1905, in Huddersfield Infirmary, Scrapbook of Press Cuttings and Miscellany, 1892–1926, West Yorkshire County Record Office (C500/5/2).

50 *Lancet*, 1910, vol. I, p. 615.

51 Ibid.; *Contemporary Biographies*, ed. by W. T. Pike, no. 6, Brighton, 1902, p. 178.

52 W. Turnbull, *An Appeal, in Behalf of the Intended Hospital at Huddersfield*, Huddersfield, n.d. [*c*.1825], Kirklees Central Library, Local History (Tomlinson Collection).

53 *The Huddersfield & Upper Agbrigg Infirmary: Laying of the First Stone*, Huddersfield, 1829, Kirklees Central Library, Local History (Tomlinson Collection).

54 *Huddersfield and Holmfirth Examiner*, 2 July 1831.

55 *The Huddersfield & Upper Agbrigg Infirmary: Laying of the First Stone*, op. cit.

56 *Huddersfield and Holmfirth Examiner*, 2 July 1831.

57 See Marland, 1987, op. cit., esp. pp. 319–22, 329–36.

58 *West Riding Herald and Wakefield Commercial and Agricultural Journal*, 15 July 1836.

59 Marland, 1987, op. cit., pp. 119, 121.

60 *Annual Report of the Huddersfield Dispensary and Infirmary, 1831–2*.

61 *Minute Book of the Huddersfield Dispensary and Infirmary*, vol. 2, AGM, 24 June 1859.
62 S. Knaggs, 'Some suggestions for diminishing the abuses of medical charities', *Medical Times and Gazette*, 1859, vol. 2, p. 367.
63 *Minute Book of the Huddersfield Dispensary and Infirmary*, vol. 2, Special General Meeting, 23 February 1863.
64 *Huddersfield Weekly Examiner*, 21 June 1902.
65 Ibid., 1 July 1911.
66 See Marland, 1987, op. cit., pp. 327–51, 357–68.
67 *Lancet*, 1910, vol. I, p. 615.
68 This lost them much popular sympathy, but presumably won them patients from the predominantly Whig middle-class electorate. The reactionism of the Huddersfield medical profession was remarked upon in the introduction to the 1834 Poll Book: 'Who does Lawyer Blackburne [the Whig candidate] represent? Why, not the Men of Huddersfield, but the Whigs, under the *haggard* form of a few Dead Body-Bill Doctors, FACTORY MONGERS, *Mushroom Merchants*, and their Myrmidons, who are *instinctively* against the PEOPLE, as the *shark* is against the herring' [their emphasis]. *A Copy of the Poll. Borough of Huddersfield, 1834*, Kirklees Central Library, Local History (B.324).
69 J. T. Ward, *The Factory Movement 1830–1855*, London, 1962, p. 39; R. Oastler, *Humanity Against Tyranny, Being an Expose of a Petition, Presented to the House of Commons, By Lord Morpeth, August 3rd, 1831 From Ten Factory-Mongers, Resident in Huddersfield and its Neighbourhood, Against Sir J. C. Hobhouse's Factories Bill*, Leeds, 1831, p. 5.
70 Minute Book of the Huddersfield Dispensary and Infirmary, vol. 3, Adjourned Monthly Meeting, 20 October 1884.
71 *Lancet*, 1884, vol. I, p. 838.
72 Ibid.
73 See Marland, 1987, op. cit., pp. 327–66.
74 See I. Inkster, 'Marginal men: aspects of the social role of the medical community in Sheffield 1790–1850', in Woodward and Richards, op. cit.
75 *Huddersfield Weekly Examiner*, 30 July 1881.
76 Minute Book of the Huddersfield Dispensary and Infirmary, vol. 3, AGM, 28 July 1871.
77 *British Medical Journal*, 1876, vol. 2, p. 65.

10

THE FUNCTION AND MALFUNCTION OF MUTUAL AID SOCIETIES IN NINETEENTH-CENTURY FRANCE

Allan Mitchell

One of the obvious lacunae in the historiography of modern France is the absence of a thorough study of mutual aid societies (*sociétés de secours mutuels*), which played a crucial part in public health throughout the nineteenth century and for much of the twentieth. Although the lives of millions were directly touched by the *Mutualité*, its complex evolution admittedly remains a 'puzzle' for historians and its social impact is still 'largely unexplored'.[1] The subtitle of a recent sketch of mutualism by one French scholar tells all: '*une histoire maintenant accessible*'.[2] Until very recently we have had nothing more than several older general narratives, collected and catalogued in the musty library of the *Musée Social* in Paris. To these have lately been added a few competent local monographs, as well as some bibliographical guides for the history of French social security. The rest, astonishingly, is silence.[3]

Although abundant source material for a detailed account of the mutual societies is available, the task is daunting. It will require either the supreme effort of a magistral *thèse d'état* or, more mercifully, a well-coordinated investigation by a team of trained researchers. Either will need to employ sophisticated computer techniques in order to generate the reliable statistics and firm classifications that are wanting.[4] In the mean time we must explore the archives with more or less astute sampling, which at least affords a glimpse of the mutual societies as they evolved in the nineteenth century. By means of such soundings, this chapter exploits three primary sources housed in the *Archives Nationales*:

1 Mutualist statutes, usually in the form of printed booklets, that contain the basic regulations upon which the societies were originally founded and according to which, presumably, they continued to function.
2 Ministerial dossiers concerning the dissolution of certain societies, especially after 1870, papers that provide an antidote to the statutes by disclosing the practical difficulties encountered by mutualism as France first began to adopt measures of public welfare under the Third Republic.
3 Governmental documents and cabinet records, which enable us to observe how the *Mutualité* emerged as an object of political discord in the *Belle Epoque* and hence as a crucial element in the struggle over social reform.

This survey, albeit not exhaustive, should make it possible to define the character of mutual aid societies and to determine the degree of their success in dealing with the social problems of nineteenth-century France.

What were mutual societies? Although no simple answer to that question could be sufficient, a representative selection of their statutes reveals the salient characteristics shared by most of these groups. Chronologically they began to appear during the late Napoleonic empire and the Restoration monarchy, thereby helping to fill a temporary void left during the French Revolution by the prohibition of religious confraternities and artisanal *compagnonnages*.[5] Geographically most mutual societies were urban, tending to cluster around centres of commerce and manufacturing in the early phase of France's industrial development. For that initial period it is possible to classify the membership of the societies according to their affiliation with a given locale, a type of patronage (such as the church), or a specific occupation. This rule had very few exceptions before 1848. Thereafter, under the aegis of the Second Empire, the societies often became multiprofessional or regional and thus less exclusive. But they never shed their character as voluntary associations of like-minded wage-earners.[6] The exclusivity of mutualism was reflected in the size of separate groups. The earliest societies were usually restricted to 50 or 60 participants, less often to 100 or 150. In time this stipulation, too, was relaxed as mutualism expanded and the societies were sometimes opened to 500 members or more.[7]

The primary purpose of a mutual society was to protect its members against the effects of illness by providing medical diagnosis and monetary indemnity. When disease led to death, the society guaranteed a decent burial service, attendance at which (except in the event of suicide) was ordinarily required of the fellow members. Some societies also offered benefits in case of industrial accidents (wildcat fisticuffs being excluded as a legitimate claim), although such incidents were problematical and frequently subject to litigation with employers who sought to evade liability. Beyond these primitive forms of sickness and accident insurance, the societies were increasingly confronted with the social problems of advanced age and permanent invalidity. Hence a few groups included a pension scheme among their promised benefits, but these were exceptional; the annual compensation to the totally incapacitated was normally well below a minimum subsistence. As a rule, that is, the mutual societies could simply not afford to grant long-term pensions. This issue, as we shall see, was later to pose the greatest challenge to the existence of the *Mutualité*.

Mutualists were expected to submit to a host of other requirements. They had first to pay an induction fee, which might vary between one and ten francs but was usually three to five francs. They had then to defray a regular monthly premium, typically, of one franc; tardiness was reason for a fine or perhaps, if chronic, for expulsion. New members were restricted in age to the years of adulthood from about 20 to 45. Some of the societies admitted younger workers in their late teens, but few accepted those over the age of 50. The explanation for this policy was frankly stated in guidelines for mutualist statutes, which admonished the societies to refuse applicants over 40 years old because 'the risk of illness is considerably augmented after that age'.[8] This tell-tale comment betrays much about the character of the mutualist movement. The original societies were not created to rescue paupers or to heal the sick, but to guard healthy and relatively prosperous citizens against the potential calamity of physical disability. Nearly all statutes made clear that membership was available only to those 'sound of body and mind' or 'of good life and morals'. Many statutes were still more specific: a medical examination was necessary to ensure that initiates were free of incurable disease, had no infirmity that might hinder labour, and did not lead a dissolute existence. It was perfectly consistent for the mutualist movement to preach a doctrine of self-help and 'prudence' (*prévoyance*), thereby distinguishing its activity from that of charitable institutions, which cared for the helplessly downtrodden.[9]

Thus the mutual society was above all an organization for stable breadwinners. Novitiates were expected to be salaried or self-employed, to maintain residence in a specified commune or to exercise a trade over an extended period, and to belong to no other mutual society. Particularly after 1848 it was common for statutes to demand that members desist from political agitation; and after 1871 they were also advised not to raise any religious issue in mutualist meetings. It has often been observed that the legalization of strikes and the development of syndicalism had the effect of separating political radicalism from mutualism. The known evidence confirms that generalization, but it suggests another hypothesis as well: both in its origins and in its residual composition the mutualist movement represented the protoindustrial mentality of artisans and shopkeepers far more than the emerging ambitions of an industrial labour force. Still less, for reasons indicated, did the societies speak for indigents, for minorities (such as foreign workers), for the permanently handicapped, or for the socially oppressed.[10]

Nor, at first, were they greatly concerned with the lot of women. It followed from all of the above that the overwhelming majority of mutualists were male, usually the ones to earn a decent wage that might enable them to meet regular monthly instalments. Before 1848 a woman ordinarily received attention from a mutual society only by becoming the widow of a member. At her husband's death, she was awarded funeral costs and perhaps granted a tiny stipend. When female workers were inducted, they were usually forbidden to participate at meetings or to belong to their society's administration. At best they were accorded a 'consultative voice'. In a very few instances women were also organized into their own mutual society; but these were likely to be ancillary to a masculine group. To be sure, after 1870 a growing number of 'mixed' societies were formed, but they invariably had a graduated (men more, women less) schedule of payments and benefits, thus reflecting the inequitable wage distribution of a labour market in which men earned at least one-third more than women.[11]

The benefits allowed by a mutual society of course depended on its financial income, which was drawn from entrance fees, monthly dues, contributions from 'honorary' patrons, and any other funds derived from donations, legacies, or investments. Although there was considerable variation, we may generalize that the earliest societies promised to pay their members an average of one to two francs daily for the duration of their unemployment due to illness. Such a stipulation, however, raised delicate questions about the length and nature of a disability. It did not guard the society against a patient who was able but reluctant to return to work. Most societies consequently came to adopt a formula such as this: a maximum compensation of one franc daily for the first six months, five francs weekly for the next three months, after which the society's executive committee would decide about any further indemnity. For those members finally declared 'incurable', a special scale would be implemented: for instance fifteen francs monthly if treated at home, ten francs if hospitalized. It is impossible to know precisely what these sums actually meant to those who received them, because the impact varied from family to family. If a mutualist had some savings and his illness was brief, the society's aid might make a significant difference. If not, the individual would soon be thrown on to the mercies of charity or public assistance with no guarantee of subsistence.[12]

Nearly without exception, all mutual societies employed their own physician. In a few instances, initially, members were allowed to consult any doctor in the commune or urban *arrondissement*. But it rapidly became apparent that the 'treating' (private) physician and the 'controlling' (mutualist) physician might disagree about the severity of an illness or injury, and therefore about the society's liability. For obvious reasons, then, it made sense for the statutes to require that the diagnosis of a family doctor be countersigned by the society's own. Additional fees for private medical care were normally declared to be outside the society's responsibility.[13]

The foregoing account should convey a general notion of how the French mutual societies were conceived by those who drafted their charters. Their inception belonged to an awkward age between the disarray of charitable institutions after the French Revolution and the passage of public welfare legislation prior to the First World War. During that long span of the nineteenth century, of course, the mutual societies were not static and did not always function as foreseen in their statutes. We therefore need to examine their evolution and to observe how they merged into the political development of France.

The history of the mutualist movement in France before 1848 is obscure. It is known that the number of societies in Paris nearly doubled after 1815 – from 140 in 1823 to 262 in 1846 – but available sources do not allow us to fix precisely the number of adherents there or elsewhere. Probably they did not exceed 100,000 adults.[14] In the eyes of the prefecture of police, mutualist groups were never beyond suspicion of harbouring insurrectionary plots. But government officials of the July Monarchy were also aware that workers were more likely to be docile if their stake in society was secure. There is little evidence, in any event, that the mutual societies came to be seedbeds of radicalism or that they contributed significantly to the revolution of 1848.[15]

In regard to the societies, among other things, the Second Republic was an interlude of confusion. But immediately after his *coup d'état* of December 1851, Louis Bonaparte moved to adopt the mutualist cause as his own and to vaunt the societies as instruments of social betterment. This decree by the 'Prince-President' in March 1852, according to his Minister of the Interior Fialin de Persigny, altogether changed the 'nature and character' of mutualism.[16] Actually a noticeable transformation was already in progress right after the uproar of 1848: mutual societies became larger and less exclusive, opening themselves to members from a variety of professions and admitting more women. Napoleon III was to encourage this development and to lend it his imperial patronage, while yet leaving the societies a large measure of autonomy in their internal administration. The emperor henceforth reserved the prerogative to appoint the president of individual societies, which were required to register their statutes and membership lists with mayors. Mutualism thus became domesticated under the general surveillance of the French prefectoral corps.[17]

The proper vocation of the mutual societies, we saw, was to insure their members against illness and, less often, accident. As the Bonapartist regime acknowledged, they were structurally ill-suited and financially unable to protect the aged and the infirm, those who demanded special care over long periods of unemployment. The imperial government therefore agreed to inaugurate a pension programme (*Caisse Nationale de Retraites*), conceived in 1850, that would assume these responsibilities 'under the guarantee of the state'.[18] This was, however, to raise serious issues about the scope of mutualist activity and the relationship between private and public institutions. Besides, this voluntary pension scheme remained woefully inadequate: to recognize the problem was not to solve it. A number of societies therefore continued to include retirement benefits in their statutes. Meanwhile, the societies received a fiscal boon through the increasing patronage of honorary members, who came to regard the mutualist movement as a constructive and gratifying form of philanthropy. The societies thus profited from the economic prosperity of the time and became, in their fashion, charitable organizations that filled an apparent need to give as well as to receive.[19]

An official report to Napoleon III in 1864 recorded these developments. Mutualism had made 'considerable progress', the emperor was told. There were currently 5,027 mutual societies in France with a total membership of 714,345. Of these, 628,786 were regular participants and 85,559 were honorary. Among the former, men outnumbered women by a ratio of more than five to one.[20] The expansion of mutualism was manifest. By the end of the Second Empire membership would approach the threshold of 1 million. If the role of the state was still limited, as was only fitting in an era of liberalism, France had none the less set foot on the path to an *Etat-Providence*. Yet it remained to establish what posture the societies would adopt in public welfare.[21]

The war of 1870 created a hiatus in the history of mutualism. Not only did many of its institutional records perish in the flames of the Paris Commune, but also the societies themselves were thrown into disorder. First their membership was dispersed and decimated in the military conflict. Then the tumultuous events in the spring of 1871 brushed them aside. Again, as in 1848, there was no indication during the Commune that the societies assumed an active part, conspiratorial or otherwise.[22]

The advent of the Third Republic did bring one significant change: henceforth, with Louis Bonaparte in exile, the societies would be free to select their own presidents. And, one might add, they would be alone to face the disadvantage that mobilized and missing members did not pay regular fees. A report on mutualist activity in 1874 gave some hint of these difficulties. The number of societies across the nation was listed at 5,748, barely above the level of the mid-1860s. Furthermore, membership was declining: the number of new societies being founded was more than offset by those dissolved, mostly because they were suffering from an insurmountable debt. In a few cases the drop could be ascribed to a fusion of two smaller societies, usually a sign of distress. Another statistical fact deserves mention here: the continued maldistribution of the societies. More than a quarter of them were clustered in and around five cities: Lyons, Bordeaux, Marseilles, Paris and Lille. Meanwhile, in remoter regions they were virtually nonexistent: the Lozère, Corsica, Cantal and Belfort had but four each.[23] So long as mutualism was conceived as a semi-private insurance agency for a restricted number of the labouring elite, the geographic factor could be considered of scant importance. But when the French republic began to contemplate the need for a national health service, predictably, that perspective would change.

By the 1880s the movement had resumed its expansion, and the first national congress of the *Mutualité* at Lyon in 1883 announced a determination to spread the gospel to every corner of the republic.[24] Although the ratio of creations and dissolutions shifted back to a positive balance, a significant number of societies continued to fail. Through an examination of such cases, for which dossiers were assembled by police and government officials, we are able to gather a variety of explanations for their persistent vulnerability.

Unquestionably the most frequent reason for the collapse of a mutual society was financial. Left to its own devices in the days before massive state subsidies, an individual society was certain to enter bankruptcy whenever its statutes promised more than its income permitted. This bind was particularly hazardous for those societies that guaranteed pensions, which might become an uncontrollable drain on their resources. One such instance was reported by the Paris prefect of police in 1884, when 'a single member had absorbed the funds in the course of a long illness'. Rather than continue their monthly payments for the benefit of only one recipient, the other members simply voted to terminate the society and to take their chances elsewhere.[25] Sometimes the grounds for dissolution were less idiosyncratic. Not infrequently older societies, whose founding dated back as far as the Restoration, attempted to reorganize after the rupture of 1870. But they soon discovered that times had changed, that they were unable to attract a sufficient number of new members, and that they were forced to disband permanently. Clearly a critical mass of participants and honorary members was necessary to make a mutual society viable. Otherwise its finances could not possibly sustain the minimal obligations prescribed in its statute.[26]

There were other problems that might cause a society to founder. In 1886, for example, a mutualist group of glassworkers in the department of the Aisne expired because their factory closed. The temporary dislocation of the war, we may generalize, was compounded by the debilitating effects of an economic slump that was bound to terminate some of the societies in this way.[27]

Another kind of difficulty, as noted earlier, derived from the inherent conflict between mutualism and the medical profession. A society in St Mandé was dissolved in 1892 because it was unable to secure the services of a communal physician. The Ministry of the Interior was informed that 'the doctors of the town of St Mandé have in effect manifested their opposition to this society, of which the objective and the organization appear to them to be contrary to their interests'. With some certainty one may translate this opaque language as a reference to the perennial dispute over medical fees.[28] Finally, with the passage of time, every society faced the demographic reality that its members were ageing. What began as a hardy band of young artisans in the 1870s was likely to become an impecunious collection of ailing and dying pensioners after the turn of the century – unless a means were found to attract new fellows in their wage-earning prime to join. Not all societies succeeded in doing so, and in that event they disappeared.[29]

True, this steady attrition affected only a minority of the mutual societies. But one must take into account that thousands of individuals were thereby left without any illness or accident coverage whatever. In the process many of them lost a sizeable portion of their savings. Even at best, joining a society constituted a gamble: if a member were incapacitated, he or she would receive at least some monetary compensation in the hour of need; but if no illness or accident occurred, all of the monthly payments over many years were sacrificed to the good of the group. And if the society collapsed, everyone lost. While these terms were acceptable for a segment of the regularly salaried citizenry, they were not ideal as the basis of a national health plan expected to serve the needs of an entire population. This was a limitation that the republican leadership was bound to confront as the *Belle Epoque* began.

The French ambition to have their nation embody the vanguard of civilization was sorely tried after 1870. The early Third Republic not only had to suffer through military inferiority and economic lethargy, but also stood by in the 1880s as imperial Germany laid the foundations of a welfare system that was to set a standard for the rest of Europe. In principle, and eventually in practice, the Germans thereby moved to adopt an obligatory national scheme of social insurance designed to protect all wage-earners and their families against illness, accident, infirmity and old age.[30]

In the liberal ethos of late nineteenth-century France, such bold innovations were scarcely imaginable. The inception of a comprehensive public health system on the German model would be possible only through a major intervention of the state into the private sphere, something that seemed totally incompatible with the *laissez-faire* character of the republic. Indeed, if anything, the drift of French politics was flowing in the other direction. After escaping from the étatist constraints of the Second Empire and the so-called 'government of moral order' (under Marshal MacMahon in the mid-1870s), successive republican cabinets had set off on a binge of deregulation in the 1880s, of which the unrestricted licensing of drinking establishments was emblematic.[31]

As a loose confederation of voluntary societies, the *Mutualité* accorded well with the French way of public life, all the more so after the enactment of a deregulatory law in April 1898 that relaxed governmental requirements for the chartering of new societies. Under this neo-liberal dispensation, mutualism flourished as never before, growing to a membership of nearly 3.5 million members by 1910. Meanwhile, with the creation of the *Musée Social* in Paris and the National Federation of Mutualists at St Etienne, the leadership of the movement signalled a new determination to lobby for political favours. Their efforts did not remain unrequited. A state subsidy was forthcoming in growing quantity, and President of the Republic Emile Loubet bestowed an official blessing by declaring himself to be 'the first mutualist of France'.[32]

These advances were celebrated by a banquet held at the Palais d'Orsay in December 1901 in honour of the chief executive officer of the mutualist movement, Léopold Mabilleau, who was awarded a medal by a delegate from the Ministry of the Interior. Mabilleau modestly attributed the growing importance of his public role to the '*élan national*' of the mutualist movement. Without wishing to dampen the evident enthusiasm of the gathering, however, former prime minister Léon Bourgeois put the French achievement into comparative perspective. Whereas the mutual societies could claim to cover 'only' 3.5 million members 'in an incomplete fashion', he noted, the British friendly societies counted 11 million participants. In Germany, moreover, 18 million people had already entered 'the path of complete insurance'. Bourgeois challenged his auditors: 'we have much to accomplish to attain the level of other nations'. Implied but left unspoken on this occasion was the elemental issue that would determine the future of mutualism: on which basis – voluntary or obligatory – would France attempt to found a social welfare system for such vast numbers of its population?[33]

An intense debate ensued, which began in intellectual circles and soon entered the political arena. We may cite as a brief for the principle of obligation a 1902 reformist tract by the Parisian barrister, Albert Crochard. He argued that France must choose between the English and the German models, 'two absolutely opposite conceptions'. Crochard estimated that half of the British labour force was protected by the friendly societies, a statistic that was laudable but still 'insufficient'. In Germany, on the other hand, fully four-fifths of workers were covered under Bismarckian social legislation; and shortly all salaried persons in the Kaiserreich were to be included. Germany provided 'an invaluable example', wrote Crochard, 'worth the trouble of attempting to imitate'. The French mutual societies, by contrast, accounted at most for one-seventh of French labour (even by a narrow definition of that term). Thus it was a 'dangerous illusion' to believe that the social question could be successfully addressed by the voluntarist solution of mutualism. Repugnant as a mandatory programme of health insurance might be to the French, Crochard concluded, the German system was undoubtedly 'the most rational and the most equitable'.[34]

An opposing argument appeared in 1904 from Léopold Mabilleau, then director of the *Musée Social* as well as president of the mutualist federation. He, too, situated France between the English and German models, but he described the French system as 'mixed', that is a distinctively Gallic combination of voluntary and obligatory features. French in origin, this solution had been adopted in other 'Latin' regions: Belgium(!), Italy, Spain and Hispanic America. Mutualism, Mabilleau contended, should be seen as 'the spontaneous product of a national instinct' born of practice rather than of theory, 'independent of the law and almost in spite of it'. This last remark introduced a harsh critique of the republic's existing public welfare service (*assistance publique*), which Mabilleau accused of squandering prodigious sums and obtaining only 'insignificant results'. The problem was that state-sponsored charity tended to undercut 'the spirit of initiative and prudence in our country'. Precisely this was the goal of mutualism, which was 'flourishing admirably' in the wake of deregulatory legislation. France must therefore encourage the extension and unification of the mutualist movement and discard proposals for a compulsory national pension plan. State intervention, Mabilleau concluded, was bound to bring the paralysis and ruin of efforts to provide viable social insurance through the mutual societies, whose prosperity depended on the immutable principles of 'liberty' and 'solidarity'.[35]

From the rhetorical duel between Crochard and Mabilleau we can easily locate the leading ideas and key phrases that were subsequently repeated in public meetings and parliamentary debates. That is another story.[36] Let it be recorded here only that the political struggle between these two positions delayed enactment of a Pension Bill for nearly a decade and that the Bill's final passage in 1910 marked a serious disappointment for mutualism. In principle, at least, it was the German model that prevailed: the law foresaw an obligatory national retirement system under state tutelage and left the future status of mutualism unclarified. As it happened, the new legislation proved both unpopular and unenforceable. Its terms had to be revised within two years by raising compensation rates and lowering the age of eligibility from 65 to 60. This trouble came as no consolation to mutualist leaders, who had hoped to gain official recognition for the movement as a corner-stone of French social welfare. Now, instead, they were faced with further uncertainty.[37]

Mutualism none the less remained a major factor in public health provision. Both its strengths and weaknesses were revealed in the process. Because these were to some extent quantifiable, it should be instructive in conclusion to consider the statistics of mutual societies on the eve of the First World War. Not only had they survived the nineteenth century, but also they had clearly experienced substantial growth since 1852 (see Table 2).

Moreover, their expansion was continuing and even accelerating in the immediate pre-war decade, despite the fact that several hundred societies were disbanded during that time (see Table 3).

While the entire movement grew, most mutual societies remained small. As late as 1910, about one-third of them still had fewer than fifty members, another third fewer than one hundred, and fewer than five hundred societies could claim more than a thousand.[38] The uneven distribution of the societies had hardly been attenuated in the nineteenth century. About 28,000 of France's more than 36,000 communes had none at all. The Paris region had gradually taken the lead: 94 per cent of communes in the Department of the Seine had at least one mutual society, followed by the Ain (70 per cent), the Pyrénées-Orientales (62 per cent) and the Rhône (61 per cent). Trailing far behind, as always, were the more rural departments of Cantal (3 per cent), Corrèze (4 per cent), Corsica, Côtes-du-Nord and Lozère (all with 5 per cent).[39]

A relatively recent innovation deserves separate mention.

Table 2 Growth of mutual societies, 1852–1902

Year	Number of societies	Membership (adults)
1852	2,488	239,501
1857	3,609	416,881
1862	4,386	565,163
1867	5,829	750,590
1872	5,793	691,241
1877	6,078	814,393
1882	7,279	1,017,225
1887	8,427	1,130,463
1892	9,662	1,288,021
1897	11,335	1,539,104
1902	13,673	2,073,569

Source: Anatole Weber, *A travers la mutualité: Etude critique sur les sociétés de secours mutuels*, Paris, 1908, p. 29

Table 3 Mutual societies created and dissolved, 1903–10

Year	Societies created	Societies dissolved	Net increase
1903	830	61	769
1904	1,019	61	958
1905	1,174	68	1,106
1906	966	48	918
1907	791	53	738
1908	730	33	697
1909	760	57	703
1910	819	54	765

Source: Yves Guyot, 'Les diverses formes de la mutualité', *Journal des économistes*, 1913, vol. 72, p. 8

Mutualism began sponsoring societies for pregnant women and young mothers (*mutualités maternelles*), a movement founded by Félix Poussineau in 1892. By the end of 1910, however, these special new societies had only 35,000 members, of which 23,000 were located in Paris alone. Mutualism, like France itself, tended to be top-heavy.[40]

It was characteristic of the societies, we should note, that they made relatively little use of the liberties offered them by deregulation. Most still preferred to be placed under government surveillance. In the two decades before 1902, membership of 'approved' societies increased by 1 million, but that of 'free' societies by only 100,000 – a proportion that remained largely unaltered.[41] The explanation was simple: state subsidies were available only under government control. Just how significant these funds were for the *Mutualité* may be gathered from a global survey of its finances (see Table 4).

Table 4 Budget of mutual societies, 1910 (francs)

Receipts		
from entrance fees and dues	39,363,515	
from donations, legacies, and		
contributions of honorary members	11,889,728	
from state subsidies	11,721,945	
Total		62,975,188
Expenditures		52,394,718
Balance		10,580,470

Source: Anatole Weber, *Les Errements des sociétés de secours mutuels*, Paris, 1913, pp. 16–25

We can recognize that without state support the mutual societies would have scarcely been able to make ends meet. Indeed, were it not for the 'extraordinary' receipts from state and private contributions, mutualism would have incurred in 1910 alone a deficit of over 12 million francs. The exactitude of these figures is not beyond challenge. But it was symptomatic that both Léopold Mabilleau and his notable ally, Emile Cheysson, came to favour a sweeping increase in membership fees in order to ensure the survival of the societies. Not only was the legal status of the mutual societies left in doubt before 1914, but also, we must conclude, their financial condition remained precarious.[42]

The story of the French mutual aid societies, in so far as it has been told at all, is usually recounted from the vantage point of the present. Seen retrospectively, mutualism can be regarded as a harbinger of the system of social security adopted by France after 1945. According to this scenario, prior to 1914 the French deliberately chose a path between liberalism and *étatisme*, hoping thereby to assuage the nation's social needs without succumbing to undue state intervention. But the First World War unavoidably enhanced the role of the state and eroded French scruples against obligatory health regulations. After some hesitation in the inter-war years, and once liberated from German occupation in 1944, the French finally moved to lay the foundations of a public welfare system worthy of the name.[43]

There is obviously much truth to this version, which no scholar would dismiss out of hand. Yet there is a different perspective on the mutual societies that is bound to become more compelling as archival researchers attempt to reconstruct their origins. Mutualism was conceived in the early stages of France's industrial growth, at a time when manufacturing and commerce were mostly the work of artisans, shopkeepers and unskilled labour. The statutes of these initial societies show that they were exclusive and defensive in posture. They were intended to preserve the status of a few, not to serve the needs of many. The day-to-day operation of the societies thereafter testified to this elitist character. Hence they were congenitally unsuited for the assignment that their own leaders eventually sought to claim for them as the purveyors of national health care. Solidarism, not socialism, should be properly associated with the *Mutualité*, whose original gospel and subsequent activity failed to reach much of the modern industrial labour force of France. It is thus fitting that the names of Jules Guesde and Jean Jaurès do not appear in this account. We read instead of Léopold Mabilleau, Emile Cheysson, and Léon Bourgeois – personalities that dominated the late nineteenth century but that seem diminished in the twentieth. Arguably they deserve to be viewed as the last of the liberals rather than as the pioneers of social security. If so, the mutual aid societies are better understood as links with the past than as forerunners of the future.

NOTES

1 B. Gibaud, *De la mutualité à la sécurité sociale: Conflits et convergences*, Paris, 1986, p. 14.
2 M. Dreyfus, *La Mutualité: Une histoire maintenant accessible*, Paris, 1988, pp. 11–13.
3 Local studies include J.-P. Navarro, *La Naissance des sociétés de secours mutuels dans le Tarn*, Toulouse, 1983; J. Y. Chalvignac, *Sociétés de secours mutuels en pays de Fougères, de la fin du Second Empire au début de la IIIe République*, Rennes, 1985; and A.-M. Guimbretière, *Racines mutualistes. Sociétés de secours mutuel vendéennes. Milieu XIXe–Début XXe*, n.pl., 1985. As guides to books and documents, respectively, see N. Dada, *Bibliographie pour servir à l'histoire de la sécurité sociale, de l'assistance et de la mutualité en France, de 1789*

à nos jours, Bordeaux, 1980; and Dreyfus, *Les Sources de l'histoire ouvrière, sociale et industrielle en France (XIXème et XXème siècles)*, Paris, 1987.

4 See the preface by Madeleine Rébérioux to a symposium on mutualism published in *Prévenir*, May 1984, vol. 9, pp. 3–5.

5 On the distant background see J. Bennet, *La Mutualité française des origines à la révolution de 1789*, Paris, 1983. On the link with confraternities of the Old Regime and the 'drift from compagnonnage to mutual aid societies', see W. H. Sewell, Jr, *Work and Revolution in France: The Language of Labour from the Old Regime to 1848*, Cambridge, 1980, pp. 163–71, 184–7.

6 As an example of each of the three types one may cite, respectively, 'Règlement de la 41me société de prévoyance et de secours mutuels des ouvriers de tous les arts dans la ville et des faubourgs de Lyon', 9 April 1843, Archives Nationales (hereafter: AN) Paris, F12 4822; 'Règlement pour la société de bienfaisance des ouvriers de Neuville-sur-Saône (Département du Rhône), fondée en 1821', 1843, ibid.; and 'Règlement d'une société de bienfaisance, composée d'ouvriers menuisiers de Toulon à établir dans les auspices et avec l'approbation des autorités', 12 May 1841, ibid., 4821. For a slightly different typology, see Henri Hatzfeld, 'Note sur la mutualité au XIXe siècle', *Prévenir*, May 1984, vol. 9.

7 One may compare, for example, 'Compte rendu de la société de prévoyance: les amies de la fidelité, fondée à Paris le 14 novembre 1824. Liste d'affiliation', 1841, AN Paris, F12 4822; 'Règlement de la société de bienfaisance et de secours mutuels de tailleurs de pierres, créée à Lyon', 1845, ibid.; and 'Société mutuelle des conducteurs de machines à vapeur [Elbeuf]', 1 January 1849, ibid., 4821.

8 Ministry of the Interior, *Sociétés de secours mutuels: statuts-modèles conformes à la loi du 1er avril 1898*, Paris, 1899, p. 3.

9 For example 'Règlement de la société de bienfaisance mutuelle pour les ouvriers fileurs formée le 27 mars 1819 [Nantes]', 23 February 1841, AN Paris, F12 4821; 'Règlements de la société de bienfaisance établie, en 1809, dans la ville de Montesquieu-de-Volvestre', 1846, ibid.; 'Société de secours mutuels La Prévoyante: règlement [Dieppe]', 1 May 1849, ibid.

10 For example 'Société de fondeurs en fer [Rouen]', 1839, ibid.; 'Société de secours mutuels entre les ouvriers tanneurs et corroyeurs: règlement [Nantes]', 5 February 1843, ibid.; 'Société philanthropique ou de secours mutuels entre commerçants et anciens militaires fondée à Thouars [Deux-Sèvres]', 8 July 1849, ibid.; 'Société fraternelle libre d'un groupe d'ouvriers galvaniseurs: règlement de la société [Paris]', 1 September 1881, ibid., 5386.

11 For example 'Statuts de la caisse des veuves et des orphelins de la société philanthropique de Thouars', 13 April 1851, ibid., 4821; 'Statuts de la société de secours mutuels à Cagnes', 26 April 1856, ibid., 5344; and 'Société de secours mutuels des jardiniers des Alpes-Maritimes: statuts', 1868, ibid.

12 For example 'Société de secours mutuels [Ancenis]', 1 April 1829, ibid., 4821; 'Société de secours mutuels entre les ouvriers tanneurs et corroyeurs: règlement [Nantes]', 5 February 1843, ibid.; and 'Règlement

de la société de bienfaisance et de secours mutuels des tailleurs de pierres, créée à Lyon', 1845, ibid., 4822.

13 For example 'Règlement de la société dite de précaution [Douai]', 1840, ibid., 4821; 'Règlement de la société formée le 27 mars 1819 [Nantes]', 23 February 1841, ibid.; and 'Société de secours mutuels entre tanneurs et corroyeurs: règlement [Nantes]', 5 February 1843, ibid.

14 See Dreyfus, 1988, op. cit., pp. 16–19.

15 See R. Lavielle, *Histoire de la mutualité, sa place dans le régime français de securité sociale*, Paris, 1964, pp. 42–8; and Sewell, op. cit., pp. 176–7, 256–65.

16 'Instruction générale pour l'exécution du décret relatif aux sociétés de secours mutuels', 29 May 1852, AN Paris, F12 4812.

17 See Dreyfus, 1988, op. cit., pp. 20–5.

18 'Avis aux sociétés de secours mutuels concernant la Caisse de retraites pour la vieillesse', 1855, AN Paris, F12 4812. This memo noted that 'a great number of mutual aid societies have perished through attempts to offer pensions that they were unable to afford'.

19 See G. Berjonneau, *Les Retraites pour la vieillesse et les sociétés de secours mutuels*, Paris, 1900, pp. 13–38, 130–4.

20 *Rapport à l'Empereur sur la situation des sociétés de secours mutuels . . . année 1864*, Paris, 1865.

21 See F. Ewald, *L'Etat providence*, Paris, 1986, pp. 208–13; Gibaud, op. cit., pp. 28–30; Dreyfus, 1988, op. cit., p. 25.

22 Characteristically no mention is made of mutualist activity by W. Serman, *La Commune de Paris*, Paris, 1986.

23 *Rapport sur les opérations des sociétés de secours mutuels pendant l'année 1874*, Paris, 1876, pp. 7–9. The greatest concentrations were located in the departments of the Rhône (247), Gironde (236), Bouches-du-Rhône (234), Seine (212), and Nord (202).

24 See Rebérioux, 'Premières lectures du congrès de 1883', *Prévenir*, May 1984, vol. 9.

25 Prefect of Police to the Ministry of the Interior, 18 February 1884, AN Paris, F12 5386.

26 Prefect of Police to the Ministry of the Interior, 15 July 1874, ibid.

27 Prefect of the Aisne to the Ministry of the Interior, 3 December 1886, ibid., 5343.

28 Prefect of Police to the Ministry of the Interior, 27 June 1892, ibid., 5387.

29 Prefect of Police to the Ministry of Labow 19 February 1907, ibid., 5386. In this instance nine of the remaining thirteen members were retired.

30 For an overview see P. Flora and A. Heidenheimer (eds), *The Development of Welfare States in Europe and America*, New Brunswick, NJ, 1981.

31 See A. Mitchell, 'The unsung villain: alcoholism and the emergence of public welfare in France, 1870–1914', *Contemporary Drug Problems*, 1986, vol. 13. For a more general view see Hatzfeld, *Du paupérisme à la sécurité sociale 1850–1940*, Paris, 1971, pp. 33–101.

32 The text of the 1898 legislation and other relevant enactments may be found in A. Nast and J. Michel (eds) *Receuil des lois, décrets, arrêts et*

circulaires concernant les sociétés de secours mutuels, Paris, 1913. Also see Dreyfus, 1988, op. cit., pp. 29–39.

33 L. Bourgeois, *Discours prononcé au banquet offert à M. Mabilleau le 20 décembre 1901*, Paris, 1902, pp. 23–9.

34 A. Crochard, *L'Assistance obligatoire contre la maladie et les sociétés de secours mutuels en France*, Paris, 1902, pp. 14–15, 222, 285–6, 290–306.

35 L. Mabilleau, *La Mutualité française: Doctrines et applications*, Bordeaux, 1904, pp. 11–15.

36 The broader political context will be provided by my forthcoming study to be entitled *The Divided Path: The German Influence on Social Reform in France after 1870*.

37 See Hatzfeld, op. cit., p. 57; Dreyfus, 1988, op. cit., pp. 39–42.

38 A. Weber, *A travers la mutualité. Etude critique sur les sociétés de secours mutuels*, Paris, 1908, pp. 40–1; and Weber, *Les Errements des sociétés de secours mutuels*, Paris, 1913, p. 35.

39 *Recueil de documents statistiques sur les sociétés de secours mutuels*, Paris, 1911 p. 2.

40 Ibid., p. 9. 'Note sur le nombre de communes possèdant une société de secours mutuels ou de retraites', 24 March 1909, AN Paris, F22 1. See Lavielle, op. cit., pp. 64–5.

41 Weber, 1908, op. cit., p. 29. Weber's statistics were taken directly from reports by the French Ministry of the Interior.

42 Rather than the 11.7 million francs of direct state subsidies to the mutual societies calculated by Weber, the figure was estimated at slightly more than 10 million by Yves Guyot, 'Les diverses formes de la mutualité', *Journal des économistes*, 1913, vol. 72. But the same generalizations hold true.

43 This is the basic plot of both leading French experts on the subject: Gibaud, op. cit., pp. 57, 92–3; and Dreyfus, 1988, op. cit., pp. 42–71.

11

THE MODERNIZATION OF CHARITY IN NINETEENTH-CENTURY FRANCE AND GERMANY

Paul Weindling

During the nineteenth century there was a shift away from a paternalistic form of welfare towards professionally administered and insurance-financed systems. The question arises to what extent the legacy of Christian humanitarianism and mercantilist concern with population numbers contained in earlier concepts of *bienfaisance*[1] and of the *Wohlfahrtsstaat* were reformulated in a more modern guise rather than rejected.[2] The financial bases of welfare expanded with industrialization, although there was no simple correlation between industrial growth and new forms of medical care on a socialized basis.[3] Democratic expectations of benefits according to need rather than on a charitable and discretionary basis meant that charity and the stigmatization of poverty were intertwined. Yet schemes for reform mooted during the 1880s and 1890s retained a place for voluntary agencies, which have survived in most welfare systems. Charity was modernized. Separate facilities were held to be necessary for the sick and for the poor; the incurable were separated from the infectious. Special measures and institutional arrangements were made for such groups as children, unmarried mothers and the aged.

The modernization of the voluntary sphere was a complex process, reflecting political and social tensions. Welfare became a battle ground between church and state, and between industry and labour; socialized medical schemes were opposed by free professionals. Rival systems of church and state hospitals and welfare institutions evolved. Ever more comprehensive systems of state welfare were supported by secularizing and politically radical forces. Conservatives clung to the virtues of discretionary charity, and socialists argued for radical economic reforms which would abolish poverty altogether.[4] But between these two extremes there was a complex range of reforming schemes involving varying elements of voluntary and state action. Such action took place within an array of highly diverse organizational structures, and historians are confronted with the task of unravelling welfare systems of labyrinthine complexity. Liberalism gave renewed impetus to philanthropic associations, and the rise of imperialist concern with social conditions encouraged co-ordination of voluntary agencies.

There continued to be a broad range of voluntary activity, despite the scientizing and laicizing trends in health care.[5] The voluntary and church sectors expanded at the same time as state welfare. The most notable French example is the *Société de Saint Vincent de Paul*.[6] This was founded in 1833 for the visiting of the poor and sick, and grew steadily during the nineteenth and early twentieth centuries.[7] German state and municipal hospitals were often staffed by religious nursing orders. Protestant and Catholic nursing orders expanded, even though there were increasing numbers of secular orders and freely practising nurses.[8] Church-based charitable organizations thrived. The German Protestant *Innere Mission* was founded in 1848, and the Catholic *Caritas* organization in 1897. Diverse political viewpoints underpinned the continuing importance of the voluntary sphere in coping with the intractable problems of burgeoning urban populations. Voluntary initiatives remained vital where it was felt the state could not or should not reach. The voluntary agencies both supplemented state welfare and demanded official approval in order to secure their continuing existence.[9]

There continued to be an administrative dichotomy between voluntary aid and the much reviled Poor Law measures. Germany and France in the 1880s and 1890s offered alternative schemes of medical assistance. How did the *assistance publique* and the French national medical assistance legislation of 1893 compare with the Bismarckian social insurance provisions of the 1880s and family welfare schemes in the 1890s? Although in both countries the state took major legislative and supervisory roles, any assumption of a unitary welfare state would be misleading. The complexity of the resulting forms of welfare may be ascribed to diverse client groups. Urban health was a major cause for concern in a period when the rate of population increase was greatest in the largest cities.

It is instructive to compare the French model of the *assistance publique* with the emergent German system of sickness insurance. This provides a contrast between a state-administered poor relief organization, and worker- and employer-financed systems. Political rights were a key feature of the French reforms, whereas the German system rewarded economic activity. While both systems aimed to integrate the working class, they each had defects and omissions. The new insurance and medical poor relief systems were both unsuited for family dependants, for maternity and for rural areas. In response to this situation, attempts were made to develop a national system of medical provision in French rural areas. Germany saw the centralization of charitable organizations for example in the cases of tuberculosis and infant welfare. Schemes for maternity benefits further illustrate divergent social trends, as there was a growth of pro-natalist concern with the family and the declining birth-rate. Both social systems reveal the importance of professional interests. Here again the situation was problematic. On the one hand the right to free medical care dispensed by professional doctors meant that workers acquired a sense of dependence on a bourgeois elite. On the other hand, doctors' organizations lobbied against any comprehensive system of medical care, which might turn doctors into employees of the state. At no stage therefore could a rationally administered and unitary welfare state emerge. Welfare remained subject to the contradictory political forces generated by feminism, socialism, liberal voluntaryism and professional autonomy, and by the expansive bureaucracies of imperialist states.

STATE REMEDIES IN FRANCE

Nineteenth-century France had a highly diverse and localized system of welfare provision. France's network of hospitals was complemented by the *bureaux de bienfaisance* which had been established in 1797 and were administered by local dignitaries.[10] These *bureaux* had varied sources of income, which derived from state and private bonds, lotteries, an amusement tax, municipal tolls (*octrois*) and the sale of cemetery plots.[11] But the most influential model of welfare provision for large metropolitan centres was that of the Parisian *assistance publique*. This was a state-administered body under the prefect of the Seine and ultimately the Minister of the Interior. Politically acceptable notables were appointed to administer the Paris hospitals, asylums, orphanages and home-care *bureaux*.[12] The *assistance publique* had been established in 1797 as the administrative authority over the Paris hospitals and further reformed in 1849. A law of 1851 obliged communes to take responsibility for their sick poor.[13] The *assistance publique* received part of its income from an annual grant voted by the municipal council of Paris. It also drew on the accumulated wealth of charitable resources deriving from earlier centuries, and maintained independent sources of income with investments in urban and rural properties, which were increasing in value.[14]

Under Napoleon III the *assistance publique* was a useful means of political patronage, providing the state with a means of dispensing honours and offices. Yet its status as a unitary system was eroded owing to rivalries in the administration of Paris. Responsibility for public health was divided between the prefect of police and the prefect of the Seine.[15] Haussmann came into conflict with rival authorities, preferring housing reform to sanitary improvements.[16] Home-relief boards (*bureaux de charité*) were a means of promoting home visiting as the basis of primary health care.[17] The *assistance publique* developed under the Third Republic as a means of state intervention in the metropolis, which, since the Paris Commune of 1870, was without a democratically elected mayor.

The Parisian *assistance publique* went on to provide the basis for a national system of medical welfare. In 1888 hospitals were placed under the control of a *Conseil supérieur de l'assistance publique*. The extension of hospital activity with neighbourhood dispensaries, and the qualitative improvement of therapy with such advances as serum therapy for diphtheria from 1894, gave rise to professional anxieties over a state system. Doctors argued for a domiciliary system of medical care. This was the policy of the *Union des Syndicats médicaux de la France*, founded in 1881, and their journal *Concours médical*. This professional trade union argued for a decentralized and professionally controlled system of Poor Law medical practice, with payment on a fee-per-service basis. There was hostility to the founding of dispensary clinics providing free medical care.[18] Preference for domiciliary care reinforced trends towards the liberal position, that voluntary provision was superior; this was of special benefit to the medical profession.[19] Demands for a decentralized welfare system administered on a departmental basis shaped the medical assistance law of 1893.[20] Rural initiatives based on voluntary participation by physicians began to supplant state-directed cantonal medical aid for the poor. This was known as the Landais system, as it was modelled on a scheme set up in the Landes in 1856, and allowed for the participation of all physicians in care for the poor.[21]

French welfare continued to be administered on a paternalistic and discretionary basis, and substantial numbers of applications were rejected.[22] But during the final decades of the nineteenth century there was much dissatisfaction with excessive centralization and state patronage. Demands were made for elected representatives, who were to oversee municipal *bureaux d'assistance*. These marked a break with the paternalistic concept of *bienfaisance*. The municipality of Paris supported democratization. At the same time it appreciated the real need filled by the dispensaries of the conservative *Société philanthropique*. The municipality therefore supported the development of a dispensary system which would integrate institutional and domiciliary care. The reformers did not wish for a centralized state model of welfare provision. Instead solidarists demanded local control, professional standards, mutualism and the organization of welfare on a co-operative basis.[23] The activities of the *assistance publique* were perceived as highly politicized and sectarian.[24] Although the Parisian model of the *assistance publique* was the basis for a national scheme of welfare administration, this did not bring the role of the private sphere to an end. In 1886 the *Direction de l'assistance publique* was established in the Ministry of the Interior under the solidarist, Henri Monod.[25] He argued for the need to retain the private sphere as being more compassionate and subtle than the 'cold' administration of public funds.[26]

The French looked admiringly over the Channel to the Local Government Board as uniting public health and welfare services under a single ministry while allowing scope for local initiative.[27] But this unwieldy compromise between local autonomy and utilitarian centralization was ill-equipped to take positive initiatives.[28] The *assistance publique* had been an important model for the Poor Law Commission of 1834 and for the Metropolitan Asylums Board in London.[29] As Himmelfarb remarks, during the 1840s British campaigns against poverty had been channelled into legislative reforms. In the 1880s the emphasis was on private philanthropies, institutions and charities.[30] By the time of the Poor Law Commission of 1905–9, sentiment had turned against the idea of a unitary state authority for all receiving public assistance.[31] Britain and France were beginning to look towards other international models, and particularly towards German insurance schemes.[32]

Two new – and related – trends were apparent in France. These were professional aspirations towards a monopoly over medical care, and public appeals for the support of laboratory research. New efforts to integrate public and private interests were expressed by the solidarist movement for a cohesive and integrated society on the basis of social justice. These demands were supported by professional administrators and doctors running public institutions.[33] They set the tone for co-ordination and co-operation between private charities and state schemes of poor relief.[34] National congresses on public assistance were held.[35] The 1892 law on the practice of medicine (*Loi Chevandier*), and the medical assistance law of 1893 marked a new concern with developing a national system of medicine geared to the needs of the poor in rural areas. It was this reform movement that was also responsible for laws in 1898 on mutual aid societies and on employer responsibility for accidents at work, providing a further stimulus to insurance societies. The 1893 legislation provided for free and universal medical aid in the home, or (failing this) in a hospital for those entitled to poor relief.[36] This law (which took effect in 1897) was biased towards the needs of rural communes and supported domestic rather than institutional care. This went with a renewed drive for professional autonomy when in 1892 the second-class physician, the *officier de santé*, was abolished as a result of professional lobbying.[37] As an effect of the law on medical services and legislation for the aged and infirm in 1905, national expenditure increased between 1890 and 1912. Numbers of *enfants assistés* rose from 95,444 in 1871 to 115,000 in 1890 but then rapidly increased to 231,337 in 1912.[38]

The modernization of charity was also evident in the founding of the Pasteur Institute in 1888. This was a privately financed institution for medical research, which also provided free treatment for rabies. Pasteur cultivated a national ethos and positive relations with state and municipal authorities as well as with private benefactors. The development of an anti-diphtheria serum in 1894 provided an opportunity further to raise the public profile of the Institute. Public appeals were made to finance the production and distribution of sera in the *bureaux d'assistance* which had just been established. Whereas previously welfare supplements were regarded as the most effective means of preventing sickness, medical research was seen as having a new therapeutic potential.[39] The Pasteur Institute provided a model which was to be emulated by the medical charities of the twentieth century. Examples are the Rockefeller Institute for Medical Research, and Paul Ehrlich's Institute for Experimental Therapy and Serum Testing at Frankfurt. Voluntary funding boosted large-scale national research institutes as science promised to remove the root causes of poverty and disease, while philanthropy was seen as merely a palliative.

GERMAN CHARITABLE ORGANIZATION AND SICKNESS INSURANCE SCHEMES

The repressive state authorities of the pre-1848 *Vormärz* period meant that the voluntary sphere provided attractive outlets for reforming activity.[40] The *Centralverein für das Wohl der arbeitenden Classen*, founded in 1844, recommended the establishing of savings banks and sickness funds.[41] There were also initiatives in workers' self-help schemes such as the *Berliner Arbeiterverbrüderung*, founded in 1849.[42] The expanding metropolis of Berlin, where new wealth and social misery were in close proximity, exemplifies the great array of charitable initiatives.[43] A pioneering crèche was established in Berlin in 1852. This was based on a Parisian model, intended for working parents.[44] The Poor Law was to some extent modernized with appointments of Poor Law doctors during the 1860s. Yet the social stigma and deprivation of civic rights which poor relief entailed meant that the state system had only limited potential. One can tentatively suggest three phases regarding the expansion of charities. First, a phase of autonomous initiatives. Second, one of national direction, as charities were grouped into patriotically oriented leagues during the 1890s. Third, a professionalized phase from the 1920s onwards, with qualified social workers and medical experts taking charge of welfare services in both the state and private spheres.[45]

The imperial constitution placed welfare outside the competence of the state, regarding it as a matter for private philanthropic initiative. Although Bismarck was concerned to use the establishment of compulsory sickness insurance in 1883 as a means of combating socialism, the administrative arrangements can be seen as being in line with the principle of a non-interventionist state. Although insurance funds were a statutory requirement for certain groups of workers, they were autonomous and self-administered organizations. The system of dual employer and worker contributions meant that they had greater resources than the *freie Hilfskassen*, which had spread from the early nineteenth century on the model of the British friendly societies.[46]

The Reich had no executive power in welfare matters other than in establishing a legal framework and monitoring developments. The federal states like Prussia did not have responsibility for welfare – only for public health as it might affect social order, for example during epidemics. Welfare was left to private associations, autonomous municipalities and local sickness insurance funds. Although associations, municipalities and insurance funds had independence from the state guaranteed by the principle of *Selbstverwaltung*, this principle of autonomous administration was subject to legal guidelines from the state. Associations – or *Vereine* – had to register with the police. Insurances were subject to joint worker and employer control, but their activities were circumscribed by state legislation and the watchful eye of the state insurance offices (*Landesversicherungsämter*).

Sickness insurance was targeted at the urban working class in large cities – those groups deemed to be especially vulnerable to socialism. Benefits were limited in size and scope. Pregnancy and venereal diseases were excluded as matters of personal moral responsibility. Family dependants of insured workers were also excluded. The appeal of socialism to women had been overlooked in the Bismarckian stick-and-carrot strategy of which sickness insurance was an essential part. The more a family-oriented mentality became a priority, the greater the realization of these defects became. From the mid-1890s certain sickness insurances began to increase the range of benefits on a discretionary basis. The *Berliner Ortskrankenkasse* exemplifies one of the larger and more dynamic sickness insurance funds which provided a range of discretionary benefits.[47]

Despite the restrictions on direct state involvement in the welfare sphere, there was a trend towards national co-ordination of charitable schemes. During the 1880s those municipalities supporting systems of out-relief for the poor co-operated with voluntary organizations.[48] The anti-alcohol movement thrived during the 1880s very much on a self-help basis. By way of contrast the tuberculosis and infant welfare schemes dating from the 1890s involved a much greater degree of patriotic ideology and direction from above. These schemes marked a reaction against what were more democratic French models of public assistance, but they had similarities to such paternalistic initiatives as the *Société de charité maternelle*.[49] Philanthropy became a national duty. This can be seen with the founding of an imperial society for the prevention of tuberculosis in 1895. While nominally a private organization, this *Central Comite der Errichtzung von Heilanstalten für Lungenkranke* had the support of high-ranking officials and aristocrats – and their wives. Its patron was the Empress, the chairman was the Chancellor and the vice-chairman was the Prussian Minister of State. It had the nationalist ethos of such patriotic organizations as the Navy League. Officials were urged to take a lead in founding local branches in a 'voluntary' capacity. The society established dispensaries from 1899. Family welfare became a focus of the campaigns against tuberculosis. Dispensaries organized home visiting, welfare measures and dietary supplements, and medical consultations. The terms *'Dispensaire'* or *'Poliklinik'* were avoided so as not to arouse the animosity of the medical profession.[50] Instead these clinics were called 'Information and Welfare Centres' *(Auskunfts- und Fürsorgestellen)*. As a result of pressure from the medical profession, treatment was not provided, but insured patients were entitled to free medical care.[51]

Although Berlin remained without a unitary municipal administration until 1920, voluntary organizations there acted as a focus for co-ordinating the activities of doctors, public health officials, municipalities and sickness insurances. This can be seen in the organization of a 'Committee for Information and Welfare Centres in Berlin and its Suburbs' under Pütter, an administrator of the central state Charité hospital. Pütter had pioneered the first dispensary clinic in Halle. Other organizers were the head of the Prussian medical department, the sickness insurance official of the *Berliner Ortskrankenkasse*, Albert Kohn, leading clinicians and medical officers. Berlin was divided into districts, each with a free public tuberculosis dispensary.[52] Family welfare was combined with the machinations of the ruling elite to maintain social status. The flexibility of the voluntary sphere meant that it was an attractive way of overcoming entrenched bureaucratic divisions in order to deal with pressing social problems.

MATERNITY BENEFITS

The dominant historical approach to the emergence of the modern welfare state lies through analysis of the embittered course of employer–worker relations.[53] Although this provides insight into employers' initiatives as well as the response of employers' organizations to the expansion of social insurance provisions, it inevitably marginalizes the issue of the family. In the sphere of family welfare, outdoor relief and private initiatives are of greater importance.

In France arrangements for infant care had long been politically sensitive. There was rivalry between the *Société des crèches* of Baron Marbeau, which in 1851 had eighteen crèches in Paris, and an officially sponsored organization under Mme Jules Mallet, which had the patronage of the Empress.[54] Benefits were the subject of political controversy at a time when feminism was an issue of increasing political importance. There was polarization between socialist schemes for working women, and conservative ideologies of the family as the basis of social order. It is therefore not surprising to find ultra-conservatives dominating the *Société philanthropique*, and being active in extending provision for postnatal care during the 1880s.[55] At the same time reforms were coming from more radical quarters. Initiatives to promote family welfare were of value in securing social integration at a time of political tension. The *Conseil supérieur de l'assistance publique* conceived of a national scheme in 1892 to promote maternal welfare with departmental maternity hospitals.[56] French solidarist politics gave a boost to schemes to protect working mothers. A pioneering infant welfare clinic was opened in 1892 by the Paris doctor, Pierre Budin, a professor of obstetrics. He had links with solidarist radicals.[57] The ensuing *gouttes de lait* movement provided an international model for the infant welfare clinic, and formed the basis for a series of international conferences.[58] Dispensaries of the Pasteur Institutes of Paris, Lille and Bordeaux provided free treatment for rabies, diphtheria and tuberculosis.

The case of infant welfare provision in Berlin reveals the importance of private schemes. This is exemplified by the *Berliner Krippenverein*, an association which established a network of crèches throughout the city.[59] This fused the ideas of Friedrich Fröbel, the pioneer of the Kindergarten, with the Parisian model of the crèche. The patriotic phase was signalled by the increasing importance of the Patriotic Women's League, the *Vaterländische Frauenvereine*. The League's initial purpose was to train women for military nursing. During the 1890s its responsibilities came to include women's welfare work. Voluntary women workers staffed many of its infant homes and dispensaries. Although socialist welfare organizations such as the Worker's Samaritan League offered a radical alternative, the Patriotic League was the largest women's organization in Imperial Germany with half a million members by 1910. Domestic welfare work such as nursing in children's homes became an important sphere of voluntary – but officially directed – activity. The crusade against infant mortality became a nationalist rallying cry.

The opening in 1909 of the Kaiserin Auguste Viktoria Haus (KAVH) for the combating of infant diseases marked a further stage in the centralization of charity. Instead of merely informal official direction, a central imperial institution was established. Although a private organization, it had the status of a privileged official body. Fund-raising was directed by leading state officials, academics and aristocrats. Carl von Behr Pinnow, who enjoyed close relations with the Emperor and Empress, played a leading part in the foundation and administration of the KAVH. The latter took a central role in the direction of infant welfare organizations, trained infant nurses, and, particularly during the hot summer months when infant mortality was high, issued public warnings on the need for domestic and personal hygiene. Pro-natalism became an increasing concern underlying many of the medical activities of the KAVH.[60] The radical alternative to the KAVH was the League for the Protection of Mothers (*Bund für Mutterschutz*). This sought to reform conditions in maternity hospitals, and took a lead in the agitation for increased availability of contraceptives and, by the 1920s, for provision of birth control clinics.

Maternity insurance exemplifies the transition from a radical political model to state direction. The concept of maternity insurance was developed by Lily Braun, a leading socialist and feminist.[61] She derived it from a French treatise, *L'Assurance maternelle* (Paris, 1897), by the feminist campaigner, Louis Frank, and two doctors, Keiffer and Louis Maingie. She reviewed this volume in the *Archiv für soziale Gesetzgebung und Statistik*.[62] The aim of maternity insurance schemes was that working women should be provided with paid leave before and after childbirth. This view arose from a concern with the general health of women workers. Frank and the other authors were influenced by German sickness insurance schemes, and they demanded that pregnancy should attract the same benefits as sickness. Lily Braun objected that instead of pregnant mothers receiving a reduced rate of pay as if they were sick, they ought to be on the equivalent of full rates of pay. She endorsed the demand for crèches, but wished them to be provided by the state rather than by factory owners. She preferred state subsidies from general taxation to a tax on those not married and on childless couples.[63]

Lily Braun's argument that the state ought to pay mothers' expenses indicates the extent to which she saw maternity insurance in the context of a socialist state. Women members of the SPD agitated for extension of insurance cover for maternity as part of a critique of voluntary philanthropy and church convalescent homes.[64] An alternative liberal but more nationalistic scheme of maternity benefits was developed by the doctor, Alfons Fischer, who was influenced by Heinrich Braun, the husband of Lily Braun. Fischer organized various small-scale schemes on a self-help basis. In 1907 he established a *Propaganda Gesellschaft für Mutterschaftsversicherung*.[65] Support came from the left liberal Friedrich Naumann, who linked maternity benefits to the issues of population policy and imperialism. Naumann's journal *Die Hilfe* combined support for feminism and social reforms with Christian moralism. This persuasive combination appealed to such public health reformers as Fischer and Alfred Grotjahn.[66] They combined health issues with concern over the birth-rate.[67]

In France the 'birth strike' was countered by massive pro-natalist campaigns.[68] The concerns of French politicians, doctors and other pro-natalist campaigners culminated in the law of 14 July 1913 for the support of *familles nombreuses* with more than three children.[69] There was much German concern that there would be a similar decline in the birth-rate. Social hygiene increasingly focused on questions of reproduction. The leading theoretician of social hygiene, Grotjahn, argued that German insurance-based schemes to promote 'child riches' were better than French schemes which were an extension of the Poor Law.[70] Pressures for improved family benefits in Germany brought about state centralization of hitherto fragmented and private initiatives during the First World War.

WELFARE AND SOCIAL INTEGRATION

The wave of Social Darwinism that was unleashed in the 1860s has conventionally been seen as antagonistic to charity and social security. Social Darwinists like Herbert Spencer argued that welfare placed excessive burdens on fit individuals.[71] Yet by the 1890s there were varieties of biologically based social ideology which emphasized altruism, co-operation and collective health instead of individualist natural selection. Commentators on the French medical assistance legislation of the 1890s emphasized the links with the solidarist ideology of national unity and social integration.[72] While Spencerian ideas of the survival of the fittest were criticized, biological concepts of the social organism and harmonic integration were used to justify state aid to the poor. Alfred Fouillée, a republican philosopher, in 1882 advocated a 'scientific' system of state philanthropy. The political economist, Paul Beauregard, who represented the sixteenth *arrondissement* of Paris and was a member of the Progressivist bloc in the Chamber of Deputies, argued that government should supplement private charity.[73] Léon Bourgeois, as head of the Third Republic's Radical Cabinet from November 1895, developed a theory of solidarism as a correction to the excesses of individualism and socialism. His tract, *Solidarité* (1896), provided the theoretical basis for seeing philanthropy and state welfare as mutually reinforcing.[74]

It is useful to compare solidarism with German organicism and British Social Darwinism. During the 1890s 'new liberalism' in Britain, and the national social movement of Naumann, marked a new consensus on the need for collectivist – but non-socialist – solutions to social ills. The fact that biology had lost much of its anticlerical tinge facilitated co-operation with voluntary organizations. New forms of biologically based collectivism were formulated during the 1890s and an attempt was made to weld together diverse social interests. This provided a new point of entry for the traditional basis of charity – the family and the church. Bethmann Hollweg, when Prussian Minister of the Interior, spoke of the need to promote the interaction of the voluntary sector with the 'organic state'. The government's function was to ensure interdependence. Solidarism was extended to pro-natalism. Solidarists supported the professionalized model of public assistance. This reinforced the trend to move away from liberal philanthropy on an individualistic basis, towards collectivist and professionalized models.

The contrast between the state and private spheres was steadily eroded. There was increasing international co-ordination in the planning of welfare systems. The first 'international' conference of public assistance in 1888 was not attended by any Germans.[75] The anti-tuberculosis and infant welfare measures from the turn of the century had high French and German involvement, although some antagonism – as over the issue of breast-feeding – was evident. The fourth international conference of public assistance at Copenhagen in 1910 had substantial French and German delegations. Imperialist concerns with the health and numbers of future military recruits, reinforced ideologies of co-operation and integration. These meant that clear divisions between the state and voluntary spheres were eroded. Each was seen as mutually reinforcing. Germany did not rely on an exclusively insurance-based system, as officials began a process of the centralization of charities. By the 1920s associations of charities – *Spitzenverbände* – were dependent on government grants. The French situation was characterized by pluralism, despite the potential for a state system of medical assistance. Although charity was modernized and its scale enlarged, it retained a place in the expanding welfare systems of the twentieth century.

NOTES

1 For *bienfaisance*, see C. Jones, 'Picking up the pieces: the politics and the personnel of social welfare from the Convention to the Consulate', in G. Lewis and C. Lucas (eds) *Beyond the Terror: Essays in French Regional and Social History, 1794–1815*, Cambridge, 1983.

2 For the *Wohlfahrtsstaat* see W. Abelshauser (ed.) *Die Weimarer Republik als Wohlfahrtsstaat*, Stuttgart, 1987; W. J. Mommsen and W. Mock (eds) *The Emergence of the Welfare State in Britain and Germany 1850–1950*, London, 1981.

3 G. V. Rimlinger, 'Welfare policy and economic development: a comparative historical perspective', *Journal of Economic History*, 1966, vol. 26.

4 O. d'Haussonville, 'Assistance publique et bienfaisance privée', *Revue des deux mondes*, 1900, 4e sér, vol. 162; J. H. Weiss, 'Origins of the French welfare state: poor relief in the Third Republic, 1871–1914', *French Historical Studies*, 1983, vol. 13, p. 58.

5 J. S. Billings and H. Hurd (eds) *Hospitals, Dispensaries and Nursing: Papers and Discussions in the International Congress of Charities, Correction and Philanthropy, Section III, Chicago, June 12th to 17th, 1893*, Baltimore, Md and London, 1894.

6 For its precursor, the Daughters of Charity, see C. Jones, 'Sisters of Charity and the ailing poor', *Social History of Medicine*, 1989, vol. 2.

7 T. Zeldin, *France 1848–1945, Volume 2*, Oxford, 1977, pp. 1016–17; C. Langlois, *Le Catholicisme au féminin: les congrégations françaises à Supérieure générale au XIXe siècle*, Paris, 1985.

8 E. Hummel, 'Zur Prägung der sozialen Rolle der weiblichen Krankenpflege bis zum ersten Weltkrieg in Deutschland', in A. Labisch and R. Spree (eds) *Medizinische Deutungsmacht im sozialen Wandel*, Bonn, 1989, pp. 141–6.

9 R. vom Bruch (ed.) *Weder Kommunismus noch Kapitalismus. Bürgerliche Sozialreform in Deutschland vom Vormärz bis zur Ära*

Adenauer, Munich, 1987.

10 Their precursors were *bureaux de charité* under the ancien régime. See O. Hufton, *The Poor of Eighteenth-Century France 1750–1789*, Oxford, 1974, pp. 159–73.

11 Weiss, op. cit., p. 50, quoting from a Ministry of Interior report of 1874.

12 J. Gaillard, 'Assistance et urbanisme dans le Paris du Second Empire', *Recherche*, 1977.

13 A. Herbert and W. Douglas Hogg, 'Paris free and paying hospitals', in Billings and Hurd (eds) op. cit., pp. 171–5.

14 J. Imbert, 'L'assistance publique à Paris de la Révolution française à 1877', *L'Administration de Paris, 1789–1977*, pp. 79–109. M. du Thilleul, *L'Assistance publique à Paris. Ses Bienfaiteurs et sa fortune mobilière*, Paris and Nancy, 1904.

15 M. Garet, *Le Régime spécial de la ville de Paris en matière hygiène*, Paris, 1906.

16 A.-L. Shapiro, 'Housing reform in Paris: social space and social control', *French Historical Studies*, 1982, vol. 12.

17 J. Gaillard, *Paris: La Ville (1852–1870)*, Lille and Paris, 1976, pp. 321–3.

18 M. L. Hildreth, *Doctors, Bureaucrats, and Public Health in France, 1888–1902*, New York and London, 1987, pp. 38–47, 77, 235, 239–43.

19 Ibid., p. 254.

20 The law was passed by the Chamber of Deputies on 12 December 1892 and decreed on 15 July 1893. Ibid., p. 270.

21 M. L. Hildreth, 'Medical rivalries and medical politics in France: the Physicians' Union Movement and the Medical Assistance Law of 1893', *Journal of the History of Medicine and Allied Sciences*, 1977, vol. 42, pp. 18–20.

22 Weiss, op. cit., pp. 53–5.

23 *Conseil municipal de Paris: Rapport au nom de la 5e Commission sur le projet de réorganisation du service des secours à domicile*.

24 Haussonville, op. cit., p. 790.

25 Weiss, op. cit., p. 59.

26 *Congrès international d'assistance*, Paris, G. Rongier, 1889. Also Haussonville, op. cit., p. 785.

27 *Congrès international d'assistance*, op. cit., pp. 267–9.

28 C. Bellamy, *Administering Central–Local Relations 1871–1914*, Manchester, 1988; for a critical view see P. J. Waller, *Town, City and Nation*, Oxford, 1983, pp. 272–80.

29 Weiss, op. cit., pp. 75–7 for comparison of Britain and France; also O. d'Haussonville, *Etudes Sociales: Misères et remèdes*, Paris, 1886, p. 12.

30 G. Himmelfarb, *The Idea of Poverty. England in the Early Industrial Age*, London, 1984, p. 529.

31 *The Break-up of the Poor Law: Being Part One of the Minority Report of the Poor Law Commission*, London, 1909, p. xii.

32 E. P. Hennock, *British Social Reform and German Precedents. The Case of Social Insurance 1880–1914*, Oxford, 1987.

33 Zeldin, op. cit., vol. 1, pp. 654–82; Weiss, op. cit., p. 59.

34 Weiss, op. cit., p. 60.
35 Ibid., p. 60.
36 Ibid., p. 62.
37 Hildreth, 1987, op. cit., p. 56; L. Groopman, 'The *Internat des Hôpitaux de Paris*: the shaping and transformation of the French medical elite 1802–1914', Ph.D thesis, Harvard University, 1986.
38 Weiss, op. cit., p. 76.
39 C. Salomon-Bayet (ed.) *Pasteur et la Révolution pastorienne*, Paris, 1986. For state hygiene see L. Murard and P. Zylberman, 'De l'hygiène comme introduction à la politique expérimentale (1875–1925)', *Revue de Synthèse*, 1984, 3 sér, no. 115, pp. 313–41.
40 H. Diessenbacher, 'Der Armenbesucher: Missionar im eigenen Land. Armenfürsorge und Familie in Deutschland um die Mitte des 19. Jahrhunderts', in C. Sachsse and F. Tennstedt (eds) *Soziale Sicherheit und soziale Disziplinierung*, Frankfurt am Main, 1986.
41 U. Frévert, *Krankheit als politisches Problem*, Göttingen, 1984, pp. 154, 172.
42 Ibid., pp. 306–14; P. J. Weindling, 'Was social medicine revolutionary? Virchow on famine and typhus in 1848', *Bulletin of the Society for the Social History of Medicine*, 1984, no. 34.
43 B. Fromm, *Die Wohltätigkeits-Vereine in Berlin*, Berlin, 1894.
44 M. Stürzbecher, *100 Jahre Berliner Krippenverein, 1877–1977*, Berlin, 1977, pp. 1–2.
45 C. Sachsse, *Mütterlichkeit als Beruf. Sozialarbeit, Sozialreform und Frauenbewegung 1871–1929*, Frankfurt am Main, 1986.
46 F. Tennstedt, *Sozialgeschichte der Sozialpolitik in Deutschland*, Göttingen, 1981, pp. 135–225; Frevert, op. cit., pp. 314–38.
47 G. Asmus (ed.) *Hinterhof, Keller und Mansarde. Einblicke in Berliner Wohnungselend 1901–1920*, Reinbek bei Hamburg, 1982.
48 R. Landwehr and R. Baron (eds) *Geschichte der Sozialarbeit. Hauptlinien ihrer Entwicklung im 19. und 20. Jahrhundert*, Weinheim and Basel. 1983, p. 146.
49 See Woolf, Chapter 6 in this volume.
50 For reports on French dispensaries in 1900 see Zentrales Staatsarchiv Dienststelle Merseburg Rep 92 Althoff AI Nr 225 Bl. 1–27.
51 P. Weindling, 'Hygienepolitik als sozialintegrative Strategie im späten Deutschen Kaiserreich', in A. Labisch and R. Spree (eds) *Medizinische Deutungsmacht im sozialen Wandel*, Bonn, Psychiatrie 1989, pp. 51–5.
52 ZSTA Merseburg Rep 92 Althoff AI Nr 230 Auskunftsstellen Poliklinik für Lungenkranke in Berlin.
53 G. A. Ritter, *Der Sozialstaat. Entstehung und Entwicklung in internationalen Vergleich*, Munich, 1989 (= *Historische Zeitschrift*, Beiheft 11, 1989).
54 Gaillard, 1976, op. cit., p. 314.
55 *Rapport de M. Le Comte d'Haussonville (Vice-Secrétaire de la Société) sur un projet de création d'asile maternel*, Paris, 1886.
56 Haussonville, op. cit., p. 791.
57 M. L. McDougall, 'Protecting infants: the French campaign for maternity leaves, 1890s–1913', *French Historical Studies*, 1983, vol. 43, p. 92.

58 D. Dwork, *War is Good for Babies and Other Young Children*, London and New York, 1987, pp. 92–102.

59 M. Stürzbecher, op. cit.

60 P. Weindling, 1989, op. cit.

61 J. Vogelstein, 'Lily Braun, Ein Lebensbild', in *Lily Braun Gesammelte Werke*, Berlin, n. d., vol. 1, p. liv.

62 *Archiv für soziale Gesetzgebung und Statistik*, 1897, vol. 11, pp. 543–8.

63 L. Braun, *Die Mutterschafts-Versicherung*, Berlin, 1906. For a survey of French schemes and legislative difficulties see McDougall, op. cit., pp. 82–9.

64 F. Tennstedt, *Vom Proleten zum Industriearbeiter*, Cologne, 1983, pp. 511–13.

65 K.-D. Thomann, *Alfons Fischer (1873–1936) und die Badische Gesellschaft für soziale Hygiene*, Cologne, 1980.

66 A. Fischer, *Die Mutterschaftsversicherung in den europäischen Landern*, Leipzig, 1911.

67 A. Fischer, 'Der Frauenüberschuss. Eine sozialhygienische Betrachtung Naumannscher Aufsätze', *Die Hilfe*, 1911, vol. 17.

68 F. Ronsin, *La Grève des ventres*, Paris, 1978; F. Thébaud, *Quand nos grand-mères donnaient la vie: La maternité en France dans l'entre-deux-guerres*, Lyon, 1986.

69 H. Harmsen, *Die französische Gesetzgebung im Dienste der Bekämpfung des Geburtenrückganges*, Berlin, 1925; A. Fischer, 'Die Erfolge der Mutterschaftsversicherung in Frankreich', *Die Hilfe*, 1907, vol. 13, pp. 5–7.

70 A. Grotjahn, *Die Hygiene der menschlichen Fortpflanzung*, Berlin and Vienna, 1926, pp. 28–9, 233–46.

71 H. Spencer, *Social Statics*, London, 1868, ch. 25 on 'poor laws'.

72 Hildreth, op. cit., p. 16; Weiss, op. cit., pp. 56–61.

73 L. L. Clark, *Social Darwinism in France*, Alabama, 1984, pp. 55, 63.

74 Ibid., pp. 67–75.

75 *Congrès International d'Assistance (Exposition Universelle de 1889)*, Paris, 1889.

12

GOVERNMENT AND CHARITY IN THE DISTRESSED MINING AREAS OF ENGLAND AND WALES, 1928–30

Bernard Harris

Historians of social policy often tend to write about the history of welfare provision as though state welfare and private charity were entirely unrelated phenomena. This tendency is particularly apparent in accounts of the history of social policy in the twentieth century, which tend to concentrate almost entirely on the development of the statutory welfare services and the ultimate emergence of the 'welfare state'.[1] Most historians would agree that the Liberal welfare reforms of 1906–11 marked a watershed in the history of welfare provision, and that after their introduction the state became the 'senior partner' in the welfare firm.[2] However, the important point about this partnership is that it was a partnership, and this means that it is important to understand the roles played by both partners if we are fully to understand the history of welfare provision.

This chapter seeks to contribute to our understanding of the history of social policy in the inter-war period by focusing on the part played by the government in the organization and development of the Lord Mayors' Fund for the relief of the distressed mining areas of England and Wales. During the inter-war period, the state worked closely with private charities in two ways. First, most inter-war governments (if not all) believed that there should be strict limits to the growth of state welfare provision, and they looked to private charity to fill the gaps and meet any 'exceptional' needs.[3] Second, the government was also anxious to make the fullest possible use of the expertise provided by private charities, and this meant that it was prepared to make financial contributions to them in order for them to provide services on its behalf.[4]

The history of the Lord Mayors' Fund provides an illustration of both these points. The Fund was originally set up by the Lord Mayors of London, Cardiff and Newcastle in April 1928 in order to provide boots and clothing for unemployed people and their families in the coalfield districts. The government was closely involved in the decision to establish the Fund, and it continued to work closely with it throughout the period of the Fund's existence. In December 1928 the government decided to make a financial contribution to the Fund and this meant that the Fund was able to continue to supply boots and clothing as well as providing supplementary feeding.[5]

By the end of the 1920s unemployment was widely regarded as Britain's major social problem. Between 1921 and 1929, the average annual figure for the total number of registered unemployed workers never fell below 1 million, and during most of this period the incidence of unemployment among insured workers was rarely less than 10 per cent.[6] However, the incidence of unemployment was not spread evenly across the whole country, and the experience of different industries and different areas varied greatly. In March 1928, when the average rate of unemployment was 9.4 per cent, the figures for individual counties in England and Wales ranged from 2.8 per cent in Leicestershire to 27.5 per cent in Carmarthenshire. The worst hit areas were the coalfields of South Wales and Durham and Northumberland: 60 per cent of the administrative districts in the coal-mining areas of South Wales and half the administrative districts in Durham experienced unemployment rates of more than 20 per cent, and in some areas more than half the insured population was out of work.[7]

The plight of the distressed areas was highlighted in a report by a special committee of the Labour Party on the economic situation in South Wales on 8 March 1928.[8] The committee found that 'there is grave unemployment and underemployment spread over wide areas of Monmouth and Glamorgan, and that in certain districts there is practically no primary employment of any kind whatever'.[9] This had a drastic effect on the financial situation of unemployed people and their families, and on the areas in which they lived. The committee found that large sections of the population were now dependent on their own savings, insurance benefits, poor relief and private charity, and in many cases both savings and insurance benefits had been exhausted. The closure of collieries had also led to a large reduction in the local authorities' rate income, and many unemployed people had got into arrears. The authorities were therefore placed in the invidious position of having to decide whether to introduce large rate increases at a time when people could not afford to pay, or to reduce the services on which they depended.[10]

The committee also examined the social impact of unemployment in the worst-hit areas. There was widespread agreement on the part of all the witnesses interviewed by the committee that many families were unable to obtain proper boots and clothing, and there was also growing evidence that the health of the population was beginning to suffer. In Abertillery, both the School Medical Officer and the school authorities claimed that 'the children were suffering from loss of "tone"', and that 'the average weight of the girls showed a distinct falling off at all ages'. The County Medical Officer for Monmouthshire also noted 'a general and progressive loss of tone among the schoolchildren'. A number of observers thought that the worst effects of the depression were being felt by the mothers. One of the Assistant Medical Officers in Monmouthshire submitted a report stating that 'the nutrition and general standard of health of the mothers has definitely deteriorated lately, and this [is] due to the industrial conditions prevailing'.[11]

In its *Report*, the Labour committee made four main recommendations. First, it said that 'steps must be taken to effect transference of population from the areas which are hopelessly derelict to other places'. Second, 'steps must be taken to liquidate the financial position of the local authorities serving the distressed areas' by means of direct government aid. Third, it called on the government to expand the existing Junior Training Centres, and to provide compulsory training for all boys between the ages of 14 and 18. Finally, it urged the government to accept public responsibility for ensuring that all children were properly clothed and fed. It said that

> the scandal of a child population without boots must be ended at once. It is not right that the provision of boots and clothing should depend solely on the self-sacrifice [of] public officials . . . or on other miscellaneous charity. . . . Public money, under public safeguards of course, must be made available.[12]

The government's response to the committee's *Report* was spelt out by the Minister of Health, Neville Chamberlain, during a debate on the Consolidated Funds (No 1) Bill in the House of Commons on 26 March 1928.[13] First, Chamberlain welcomed the committee's support for industrial transference, and pointed out that the government was already pursuing policies of this kind through the recently established Industrial Transference Board.[14] Second, he denied that the machinery of local administration was breaking down in any way. He said that

> it would be a mistake to say that the local authorities have been cowed by the difficulties they have found. My information is that [there has never] been so keen an interest in local government in these districts, or so high a level of administration as has been reached during the present trouble.[15]

Third, he also denied that there was any need for public money to provide boots or clothing for the children of unemployed miners. He told the Commons that he saw no reason why the money should not come from 'private benevolence'. Ever since the First World War, he had been astonished by the way in which 'private people have come forward and contributed to every fund where an appeal has been made for the purposes of charity on behalf of poor people', and he was certain 'that there is plenty more money where that came from'.[16]

During his speech, and throughout the whole of the debate which followed it, Chamberlain gave no indication as to whether the government intended to launch its own appeal, or whether it would encourage others to do so. However, there were at least two other major appeals in contemplation. First, Mrs Snowden was proposing to launch an appeal in conjunction with the Lord Mayors of London and Cardiff;[17] and second, the editor of *The Times* was also planning to launch a separate appeal for the relief of distress in South Wales, Durham and Northumberland. In addition, the King and Queen had been invited to attend a charity concert at the Royal Albert Hall on 22 April 1928 in order to raise money 'for the relief of underfed women and children in [the] North and South Wales'.[18]

These appeals were discussed by a special meeting at the Ministry of Health on 30 March. The President of the Board of Education, Lord Eustace Percy, said that he doubted whether the Lord Mayors' appeal would be particularly effective because it would be impossible to confine it to any one area, and in any case he did not think that the Lord Mayor of London, who would be expected to play a leading role in the appeal, was particularly enthusiastic. He thought that the proposed appeal by the editor of *The Times* would be more valuable, because *The Times* could confine itself to the most depressed areas. The Minister of Health, Neville Chamberlain, said that 'he doubted whether there really was a case for a general appeal in England for help to Wales in particular', but he thought it would be a good idea to have one 'in view of what had been said in the debate on the Consolidated Fund Bill'. In addition, he also thought that 'if a successful appeal were made, it would take the wind out of the sails of the political agitation and would help to create good feeling'. He therefore liked the idea of an appeal by the editor of *The Times*, but he thought that an appeal by the Lord Mayors would be 'inappropriate'.[19]

The meeting then went on to discuss the terms of the appeal which either the editor of *The Times* or the Lord Mayors of London and Cardiff ought to make. Lord Percy said that he had already had a discussion with the Lord Mayor of London, and had made arrangements to have lunch with the editor of *The Times* once the meeting was over. He told the meeting that he had 'advised the Lord Mayor not to touch general adult relief, but to confine his appeal to boots and clothing for schoolchildren, the feeding and clothing of expectant mothers, and assisting the transfer of juveniles and their families to places where employment could be had'. Chamberlain argued that the last point had important implications for the government's own transference scheme, and was best avoided. He thought that 'it would be convenient if the limelight was thrown on the question of boots and clothing, and the rest of the appeal left rather nebulous'. These comments were echoed by the government's Chief Medical Officer, Sir George Newman, who was particularly anxious to avoid any reference to the question of school feeding. He suggested that

> as the provision of meals had not yet been started in emergency form in South Wales and Durham ... it would be better to avoid admitting that the ordinary machinery was breaking down, as would be the case if the appeal was made to include feeding.[20]

These discussions show that the government was closely involved in the decision to launch the Lord Mayors' Fund, but they did not mark the end of its involvement. During the first seven months of the Fund's existence, over £90,000 was raised, and this money was used to provide boots and clothing for women and children and to facilitate the transfer of over 1,400 boys to areas where employment was better. In addition to this, a number of other organizations launched separate appeals of their own, and various towns and parishes made arrangements to 'adopt' mining districts in order to send relief to them.[21] However, despite these efforts, it was clear that much more needed to be done to co-ordinate the work of the various relief agencies, and that a great deal more money was also required to help unemployed people through the winter months. As a result, the Lord Mayor of London, Sir Charles Batho, and his successor, Sir Kynaston Studd, decided to relaunch the Fund on 2 November 1928. They promised that 'the existence of the Fund will not divest any public or other authority of its recognised duty or responsibility; but something more than mere compliance with legal obligations is essential if deep suffering and distress are to be avoided'. They also announced that they intended to convene a meeting of the Lord Mayors and Mayors of England and Wales towards the end of November 'for the purpose of organising a national effort to obtain a Fund adequate for the object of the appeal, and to take steps to cooperate with other schemes having similar objects'.[22]

At the same time, the government was also coming under renewed pressure from Members of Parliament (MPs) on all sides of the House of Commons to take further action to ease the distress in the mining areas. On 3 December George Lansbury pressed the Prime Minister to 'appoint a Committee of this House to consider whether it is not possible to devise some means of bringing more generous assistance to the unemployed of the country'.[23] Lansbury pointed out that the government had recently introduced a series of changes in the unemployment benefit regulations which made it much harder for unemployed people and their families to obtain statutory relief.[24] On 4 December Margaret Bondfield introduced a Private Member's Bill with the support of all the women MPs in the House, calling on the government to provide public funds for the purchase of boots for children in the necessitous areas.[25] On 5 December Ellen Wilkinson took advantage of the adjournment debate to urge the government to make a Treasury grant for the purchase of clothing. She urged the government to accept the fact that charity could hope to touch only the fringe of the problem, and that even then it could do so in only a few selected areas.[26]

In addition, the government was also coming under pressure from its own medical advisers. At the beginning of November

the Ministry of Health asked Sir Arthur Lowry and Dr James
Pearse to visit the coalfields of South Wales and Monmouthshire
in order to assess the impact of unemployment on the health
of the local population.[27] They were unable to find any clear
evidence of widespread malnutrition, or of any increase in the
amount of sickness or ill-health that could definitely be related
to poverty, but they did observe that many women were 'anaemic
and neurotic', that the number of cases of rickets had increased, and
that recovery from childbirth was 'slower than in ordinary times'.
They also found that the diets consumed by unemployed people
and their families were well below existing dietary standards. In a
memorandum on 5 December, Sir Arthur Lowry said that the diet
was deplorable, and 'except in the face of facts it would be incredible
that a family can exist in health on it week after week for prolonged
periods'.[28]

The increasing volume of distress meant that the government
was forced to take further action in connection with the distressed
areas. On 6 December the Permanent Secretaries of the Board
of Education and the Ministry of Labour held a meeting with
a representative of the Lord Mayor of London to discuss the
possibility of further co-operation between the government and
the Lord Mayors' Fund. The most important decision reached at
the meeting was the appointment of Mr Noel Curtis-Bennett of
the Civil Commissioner's Department as the Fund's Organizing
Secretary. It was agreed that Curtis-Bennett's functions would be
'to assist the Lord Mayor's staff and keep the work of the Fund in
touch with the departments of government concerned'. In addition,
the meeting also decided that the Home Secretary and the President
of the Board of Education should launch a further appeal, together
with the Lord Mayor of London, for more money to aid relief
work.[29]

The government's decision to appoint Curtis-Bennett was widely
supported, but it did not solve the financial problems of either the
Lord Mayors' Fund or the people it was set up to help, and it soon
became clear that the government would have to make its own
contribution to the Fund if it was to retain credibility.[30] Some of
the government's closest advisers believed that it should make an
immediate donation of up to £750,000 to the appeal in order to
demonstrate its concern for the distressed areas, but others felt that
a government contribution of this sort would simply discourage
private donations. As a result, the government decided instead to

donate a pound for every pound donated by members of the public. In addition, it also agreed to make a retrospective grant of £150,000 to match the amount of money which the Fund had already received since the beginning of April.[31]

The government's decision to channel relief through the Lord Mayors' Fund was welcomed by the Fund's local organizers, and by sections of the local press. When the Prime Minister made his announcement, the Cardiff *Weekly Mail* said that the government's 'lavish aid', together with the interest and patronage of the Prince of Wales, had given the Lord Mayors' appeal 'a national status and authority', and the act of contributing to the Fund had now become 'a personal and universal obligation'.[32] The *North Mail and Newcastle Chronicle* said that the decision to make an immediate grant of £150,000 was an indication of the government's 'recognition of the urgency of the need', and that the introduction of the pound for pound scheme was 'a general provocation to personal charity'.[33] However, others were rather more sceptical. The Labour Party thought that the government's contribution to the Fund should be based on an assessment of the community's needs, instead of being made conditional on the vagaries of private charity.[34] The *South Wales Daily Post* thought that the government's action might bring some temporary relief over Christmas, but it warned that 'relief will have to be continued for a long period until the slow re-absorption of the unemployed through the operation of the permanently ameliorating remedies that are being applied takes effect'.[35]

The government's decision to contribute to the Fund also meant that it became much more closely involved in the administration of the Fund and the distribution of its resources. One of the first questions which needed to be considered was whether those charities which were already working in the same areas as the Lord Mayors' Fund should be allowed to transfer their own funds to the appeal in order to qualify for the government grant. If the government allowed these organizations to transfer money, the size of the Exchequer contribution might end up being a great deal more than was originally intended, but if the organizations were not allowed to transfer money, the public would stop donating money to them, and the government would stand accused of undermining charities which had a long and honourable record of service to those in need.

The government's response to this dilemma was based on a series of anonymous memoranda which were drawn up shortly after the Prime Minister made his statement to the House of Commons.[36] The author of the memoranda identified two different types of charity which needed to be considered. The first consisted of those organizations which had made appeals for general relief on the same grounds as the Lord Mayors' own appeal; the author argued that these organizations should be allowed to transfer money to the Lord Mayors' Fund, so long as they accepted that the Fund thereby gained control over the way in which the money was subsequently distributed. The second type of organization was one which had appealed for help in connection with activities which lay beyond the scope of the Lord Mayors' appeal, such as allotments, boot-repairing shops, transference (*sic*) and emigration. These organizations should also be allowed to pay money into the Lord Mayors' Fund, but it would then be paid back to them, together with a matching grant from the government.[37]

In addition, the same author also prepared a separate memorandum on the question of those organizations and areas which had 'adopted' towns and villages in the distressed areas.[38] He (or she) was personally opposed to the practice of adoption because the adopting areas were unable to raise enough money to meet all the needs of the areas they adopted, and because the multiplicity of adopting areas was an obstacle to the efficient co-ordination of relief work. However, the practice could not be ignored because 'it appeals to the sentimental side of the public; it has received the blessing of the Prime Minister; and it focuses the interest of the contributors on an identifiable spot in a wilderness of relief'.[39] In view of the popularity of adoption, adopting organizations should be allowed to pay money into the Lord Mayors' Fund in order to qualify for the government grant, subject to the following conditions: the adopted area had to be situated in a district covered by the Fund; the money had to be distributed through the Fund's local committees; it must be used for general relief purposes; and the Fund would not be obliged to spend the whole of the government's contribution in the adopted area.[40]

The second major question which the government needed to consider was whether the Lord Mayors' Fund should be extended to cover areas outside South Wales, Durham and Northumberland. When the Lord Mayors' Fund was originally launched, the Lord Mayors placed no restrictions on the coalfields for which the money was intended, but it was generally assumed that all the money would be spent in South Wales and the north-east of England, and this assumption was borne out by events. However, once the Fund had been relaunched on 2 November 1928, a growing number of people began to argue that the Fund should now be extended to other distressed mining areas. When the House of Commons debated the introduction of the government grant on 20 December, many MPs claimed that their areas were in just as much need of help as South Wales or Durham and Northumberland,[41] and many of the local dignitaries who had been asked to co-ordinate the appeal for funds made it clear that they would give their help only if their own areas were also permitted to benefit.[42] In response, the government was forced to agree that the money which was donated to the Lord Mayors' Fund would be used to relieve distress throughout the coalfield areas.[43] This decision was announced by the Lord Mayor of London in a statement issued to the press on 11 January 1929.[44]

The announcement of the pound for pound scheme also meant that the government was forced to take a much closer interest in the way in which the resources of the Lord Mayors' Fund were actually spent. Before the Prime Minister made his announcement, the Fund had not provided any services which were already provided by public authorities, but the government's decision to use the Fund for school feeding meant that both the Fund and the local education authorities were directly involved in the provision of meals to hungry schoolchildren. This created two particular problems. First, it meant that some local education authorities might choose to abandon their own school feeding programmes in order to throw the whole burden on to the Lord Mayors' Fund; and second, it meant that the government might be appearing to reward those authorities which had been unable or unwilling to provide school meals in the past at the expense of the more diligent authorities.

These problems were discussed by a special Interdepartmental Liaison Committee on 17 December 1928 and a further discussion took place at a meeting in Cardiff on 21 December.[45] The government and the managers of the Fund agreed 'that each area must be responsible in the future, as they have been in the past, for the feeding of the necessitous schoolchildren to the extent that they have carried out that duty in the past', but they also recognized that some local education authorities had shown a much greater willingness to engage in school feeding than others.[46] They therefore decided that where the Committee of the Lord Mayors' Fund acts as the School Canteen Committee some contribution shall be asked from the local education authority, and this contribution shall be assessed with special regard to the amount that the authority have been able to do up to the present, and in some cases would not exceed or might be less than that amount.[47]

When the Minister of Health made his initial announcement about the organization of relief in the distressed areas, both the Labour Party and the Miners' Federation of Great Britain responded bitterly. The Labour MP for Bishop Auckland, Ben Spoor, said that the minister's speech was 'from every point of view a disappointing speech',[48] and the *Miner* said that it showed the government's 'complete indifference to the sufferings of the workers'.[49] However, by the end of September the volume of distress had become so great that the miners were forced to issue an appeal of their own, and when the government announced the introduction of the pound for pound scheme the Federation decided to transfer its own funds to the Lord Mayors' Fund in order to take advantage of the government grant. During the course of the following months, the miners continued to call for 'remedies not relief', but they were also extremely grateful for the help which the Lord Mayors' Fund was able to give them. Shortly after the appeal was closed, the miners' secretary, Arthur J. Cook, wrote:

> Now that the Lord Mayors' Fund has been closed, temporarily at any rate, I feel sure I am voicing the opinions of our members in thanking the Lord Mayor and those who have helped in the collection of funds, clothes etc. for the distressed miners. While we are anxious for remedies and a new order of society, we shall not be doing our cause harm by rendering proper thanks to those who have shown real sympathy to us in our distress. The Committees in the local areas must see to it that the surplus is distributed to the best advantage. While the Fund has not been adequate to meet all that we should desire, it has brought some joy to our people in the distressed areas.[50]

The Lord Mayors' Fund for the relief of the distressed mining areas was formally closed on 30 April 1929. Over the course of the previous thirteen months, the Fund had succeeded in raising a total of £1,746,841 6s. 2d., including the government grant. Just over half this money was spent on the provision of boots and clothing. The

Fund spent £340,000 on boots and clothing in South Wales, £288,000 in Durham and Northumberland, and £92,000 and £115,000 in Lancashire and the West Riding of Yorkshire respectively. The remainder of the money was shared between the coalfields of the West and East Midlands, Cumberland, Gloucester, Somerset and the Forest of Dean, North Wales and the North Riding of Yorkshire.

The second major area of expenditure concerned the provision of outfit grants for people returning to work after long periods of unemployment. The Fund spent £389,000 under this heading. Once again, the greater part of the money was spent in South Wales and Durham and Northumberland. The Fund spent just over £280,000 on outfit grants in South Wales and just over £100,000 in Durham and Northumberland. The remaining part of the money was distributed in the North and West Ridings, and in Gloucester, Somerset and the Forest of Dean.

The third major item of expenditure was expenditure on supplementary feeding. The Fund spent £90,545 on the distribution of food vouchers, and £32,060 on school meals. The distribution of food vouchers was confined to just three coalfields. The Fund spent £65,000 on food vouchers in South Wales and £22,000 in Durham and Northumberland, and the remainder was spent in the West Riding of Yorkshire. South Wales and Durham and Northumberland were the only areas to receive any help with school feeding. The Fund contributed £19,756 to the cost of school feeding in South Wales and £12,304 in Durham and Northumberland.[51] In 1929 the Chief Medical Officer of the Board of Education, Sir George Newman, reported that the Lord Mayors' Fund had enabled the local education authorities in Durham and Northumberland to feed 12,673 more children than they had been able to feed previously.[52]

The main aim of this chapter has been to examine the part played by the government in the decision to launch the Lord Mayors' Fund, and to show how the persistence of distress forced the government to become much more closely involved in the administration and finance of the Fund over the following months. When the government first discussed the problems of the distressed areas in March 1928, it argued that there was no reason why the needs of the local communities could not be met by private benevolence. However, as the degree of distress intensified, it became increasingly apparent that private charity was unable to meet the need for relief, and the government came under mounting pressure to take over the administration of the Fund and make a substantial contribution to its resources. In December 1928 the government agreed to donate a pound for every pound donated by members of the public, and this meant that it became much more closely involved in both the management and the distribution of the Fund's resources.

However, the history of the Fund also provides a vivid indication of the limitations of this policy. When the President of the Board of Education announced the details of the pound for pound scheme to the House of Commons on 20 December, he said that the position in the distressed areas was an abnormal one, and that 'it is perfectly in line with the recognised social reform legislation of this country that you should meet such an abnormal situation, not by the giving of 100 per cent grants . . . but by having cooperation' between the state and private charity.[53] However, although the situation in the distressed areas was abnormal, it was also deep-seated, and by the end of 1929 many of the problems which had led to the establishment of the Lord Mayors' Fund had reasserted themselves. On 5 December 1929 a deputation from the Standing Joint Committee of Infant Welfare Officers told the Labour Minister of Health, Arthur Greenwood, that 'the general position in South Wales was that the relief derived from the Guardians and from charitable sources had proved wholly insufficient to meet the needs', and a member of the Coalfields Distress Committee in South Shields said that in her area the money provided by the Fund 'was not sufficient to meet even half the distress'. Dr Marion Philips MP told the minister that the Fund was now practically exhausted, and that it was unlikely that any further appeals for funds would be successful.[54]

In addition, the establishment of the Lord Mayors' Fund also posed problems for other groups who were dependent on charitable support. In 1947 Constance Braithwaite wrote that 'the amount given in charity seems to have varied surprisingly little [during the interwar period] . . . if we consider all the concurrent changes in economic circumstances and public social policy which might have been expected to affect it'.[55] However, this judgement takes no account of changes in the distribution of charitable donations between one year and the next. In March 1929, when the Lord Mayor of London announced his decision to close the Fund, he said that one of his reasons for doing so was that 'the generous flow of subscriptions to this Fund cannot have been without an adverse effect upon many other deserving funds depending for their support upon private contributions'. He went on to say that he could not be expected to keep the Fund open indefinitely because 'circumstances may arise at any moment which might make it desirable for a fresh Mansion House Fund to be opened for some other purpose'.[56]

Although the Lord Mayors' Fund was officially wound up in the spring of 1930, the populations of the distressed areas continued to experience very high levels of unemployment throughout the 1930s. The government was forced to recognize that emergency appeals to private charity were unlikely to raise enough money to make any real difference to the lives of people in need, but in spite of this its own measures to help alleviate distress had only a limited effect. In 1932 the government's Chief Medical Officer, Sir George Newman, said that the combined efforts of both public and voluntary welfare agencies had ensured that despite high levels of unemployment there had been no general deterioration in health standards, but the most that can be said is that government action enabled unemployed people and their families to maintain standards of health which were already very low.[57] These standards began to show signs of a significant improvement only towards the end of the 1930s and the coming of the Second World War.[58]

Acknowledgements

I should like to thank Elizabeth Peretz, Rodney Lowe, Colin Jones, Jonathan Barry and an anonymous referee for their help and advice.

NOTES

1 See for example P. Thane, *The Foundations of the Welfare State*, London, 1982; D. Fraser, *The Evolution of the British Welfare State*, London, 1984; A. M. Rees, *T. H. Marshall's Social Policy*, London, 1985.
2 D. Owen, *English Philanthropy 1600–1960*, London, 1964, p. 527.
3 See for example *Parliamentary Debates*, 5th series, vol. 223, cols 3378–9 (comment by Lord Eustace Percy).
4 For example the government and local authorities made substantial contributions to voluntary organizations to enable them to provide voluntary hospitals and maternity and child welfare centres. See S. M. Herbert, *Britain's Health Services*, Harmondsworth, 1938, pp. 111–22; V. Creech-Jones, 'The work of voluntary social services among children before school-leaving age', in H. A. Mess *et al.*, *Voluntary Social Services since 1918*, London, 1947, p. 109.
5 The fullest account of the history of the Fund is to be found in the *Interim Report of the Lord Mayors' Fund for the Relief of Women and Children in Distressed Mining Areas*, 1929. A draft copy of this Report can be found in PRO MH 79/304. The Central Joint Committee for the Administration of the Lord Mayors' Fund also produced a second

Interim Report in March 1931. A copy of this Report, entitled *Lord Mayors' Fund for the Relief of the Distressed Mining Areas in England and Wales*, can be seen in the Guildhall Library, London (ref. SL 31/82). For details of the Lord Mayors' original appeal, see *The Times*, 3/4/28, p. 16, col. a, 'The stricken coalfields: a national appeal'.

6 C. H. Feinstein, *National Income, Expenditure and Output of the United Kingdom, 1855–1965*, London, 1972, Table 128.

7 *The Times*, 27/3/28, p. 16, col. b, 'The black areas'.

8 The committee consisted of Rhys Davies MP, F. W. Pethwick-Lawrence MP and Herbert Evans.

9 PRO ED24/1391, Labour Committee, *Report*, p. 11.

10 Ibid., pp. 5, 11.

11 Ibid., pp. 2, 6, 11.

12 Ibid., p. 12.

13 *Parliamentary Debates*, 5th series, vol. 215, cols 825–950.

14 Ibid., cols 845–6.

15 Ibid., cols 843–4.

16 Ibid.

17 I assume this was Ethel Snowden. She was a prominent member of the Labour Party and other national organizations, including the Board of Governors of the BBC and the National Education Association. She was married to Philip Snowden, who served as Chancellor of the Exchequer in the Labour governments of 1924 and 1929–31. For further biographical details, see *Who Was Who*, London, 1947, vols 3 and 5.

18 PRO ED 24/1391, Report of a meeting . . . held on 30 March 1928.

19 Ibid.

20 Ibid.

21 In December 1928 a government official wrote 'the definition of "adoption" is infinitely variable', but in the majority of cases a town or organization could be said to have adopted another town if it agreed to raise funds for the specific benefit of the adopted area. At the time this memorandum was written, the following towns and parish organizations had agreed to adopt mining areas in South Wales and Durham and Northumberland: Eastbourne (Rhymney); Worthing (Brynmawr); Willesden (Nantyglo and Blaina); St Martin-in-the-Fields (Mountain Ash); Tunbridge Wells (the Afan Valley from Aberavon northwards); Enfield (Abergwynfi and Blaengwynt); Caterham (Caerphilly); Margate (Swansea colliery area); Deptford (Ushaw Moor); St Michael's parish, Chiswick (parish of Graig, Pontypridd); Kingston and Surbiton (Seaton Burn); Upper St Leonard Parish and the Hastings and Bexhill Social Service Centre (Nantyglo); Harpenden (Risca); Wootton-under-Edge (Rhymney); Malvern Wells Rural Deanery (Aberaman); Woodford Green (Blaenavon). In addition, the *Spectator* adopted the town of Aberdare. See PRO MH 79/304, Memorandum on adoption.

22 *The Times*, 2/11/28, p. 14, col. d, 'The stricken coalfields'. The meeting of Lord Mayors and Mayors took place in the Mansion House in London on 5 December. See *The Times*, 6/12/28, p. 11, cols a–c, 'Distress in the coalfields'.

23 *Parliamentary Debates*, 5th series, vol. 223, col. 977.
24 Ibid., cols 977–8. The government had reduced the number of grants for public works; the regulations governing uncovenanted benefit for the long-term unemployed had been tightened up under the Unemployment Insurance Act of 1927; and poor relief for able-bodied men had been severely curtailed.
25 Ibid., cols 1029–32.
26 Ibid., cols 1351–6.
27 PRO HLG 30/63, Memorandum by Sir Arthur Robinson, 1/11/28.
28 PRO ED 24/1391, Memorandum by Sir Arthur Lowry. The government published a full report on the visit in 1929. See PP 1928–29 Cmd 3272 viii, 689, *Report on Investigation in the Coalfield of South Wales and Monmouth*. Lowry's comment on the diet of unemployed families raises important questions about the relationship between dietary deprivation and health standards in the inter-war period. These are discussed in more detail in B. Harris, 'Medical inspection and the nutrition of schoolchildren in Britain, 1900–1950', Ph.D thesis, University of London, 1989, pp. 118–51.
29 PRO HLG 30/63, 'Distress in South Wales, Durham and other areas', 6/12/28. The Prime Minister announced the details of Curtis-Bennett's appointment to the House of Commons on 10 December. See *Parliamentary Debates*, 5th series, vol. 223, col. 1696.
30 See for example 'Federationist', 'Generous gifts to the Relief Fund, but nothing from the Government', *Miner*, 15/12/28, pp. 2–3.
31 PRO HLG 30/63, 'Relief of distress in mining areas', 11/12/28; *Parliamentary Debates*, 5th series, vol. 223, cols 2609–10.
32 *Weekly Mail* (Cardiff), 22/12/28, p. 6, col. 2, 'Prince of Wales' call to the nation'.
33 *North Mail and Newcastle Chronicle* (Newcastle upon Tyne), 18/12/28, p. 9, cols 1–2, 'Government aid for distressed areas'.
34 See for example *Parliamentary Debates*, 5th series, vol. 223, col. 3284 (MacDonald).
35 *South Wales Daily Post* (Swansea), 18/12/28, p. 6, cols 1–2.
36 There were four of these memoranda in all, dealing with the questions of adoption, donations to other organizations, the definition of 'distressed mining areas', and the position of the voluntary organizations in the administrative structure of the Lord Mayors' Fund. They were unsigned and undated, but the internal evidence makes it fairly clear that they were written some time between 18 December and 31 December 1928. See PRO MH 79/304, Memoranda.
37 PRO MH 79/304, Memorandum on funds of voluntary organizations.
38 See note 21.
39 Ibid.
40 Ibid.
41 See for example *Parliamentary Debates*, 5th series, vol. 223, cols 3303, 3345–6, 3348, 3362, 3364, 3380–1, 3396–401, 3405–6.
42 See PRO ED 24/1391, Sir Arthur Hazlerigg (Lord Lieutenant of Leicestershire) to N. Curtis-Bennett, 14/12/28.

43 The only exception was the Kent coalfield. The government and the Fund's managers argued that Kent was not a distressed mining area because the incidence of unemployment in the region was minimal. See MH 79/304, Notes on distress and unemployment (n.s., n.d.).

44 PRO ED 24/1391, Coalfields Distress Fund – Lord Mayor's statement on administration. See also *The Times*, 12/1/29, p. 7, cols a–b, 'The distressed areas: scope of Lord Mayors' Fund'.

45 The Interdepartmental Liaison Committee met three times between 17 December 1928 and 1 January 1929. It was chaired by Lord Eustace Percy, and included representatives of the Board of Education, the Ministry of Health and the Ministry of Labour. The meeting at Cardiff on 21 December was attended by the local organizers of the Lord Mayors' Fund in South Wales. Percy Watkins attended the meeting on behalf of the Board of Education. See PRO ED 24/1391, Minutes of the first meeting of the Interdepartmental Committee ... on 17 December 1928; and ibid., Mining Areas Relief Fund, Conference held at City Hall, Cardiff, 21/12/28.

46 Under the Education Act 1921, local education authorities were empowered to make arrangements for the feeding of children who were 'unable by reason of lack of food to take full advantage of the education provided for them', but they were under no obligation to do so. In the year ending 31 March 1928, 132 local education authorities (out of 315) provided school meals. The total number of children fed was 123,677, and the total number of meals was 15,875,340. See *Health of the Schoolchild 1928*, London, 1929, p. 73.

47 PRO ED 24/1391, Minutes of the first meeting of the Interdepartmental Committee ... 17/12/28; Conference at City Hall, Cardiff, 21/12/28.

48 *Parliamentary Debates*, 5th series, vol. 215, col. 857.

49 *Miner*, 31/3/28, p. 8, col. d, 'The plight of the coalfields'.

50 *Miner*, 4/5/29, p. 4, col. b, 'The Secretary's Review'.

51 The closure of the Fund was announced in *The Times* on 27/3/29. See p. 15, col. c, 'Closing the Fund'. There is a preliminary statement of the Fund's accounts in PRO ED 24/1391, Analysis of grants, 18/3/30. Full details of the total expenditure by the Fund and its local committees are given in Guildhall Library SL 31/82, *Lord Mayors' Fund for the Relief of the Distressed Mining Areas in England and Wales*, pp. 72–101.

52 *Health of the Schoolchild 1928*, p. 71.

53 *Parliamentary Debates*, 5th series, vol. 223, col. 3378.

54 PRO ED 24/1391, Report of a meeting between the Minister of Health ... and a deputation from the Standing Joint Committee of Infant Welfare Officers, 5/12/29. See also PRO MH 57/97D, 'Report of Mr James Evans on District 14, covering 53 Unions in Wales and Monmouthshire'. Evans wrote: 'The institution of the Lord Mayors' Fund and the commendable efforts made by the Society of Friends and other agencies in the provision of work schemes and the establishment of clubs and centres of recreative and intellectual pursuits are doing something to mitigate the serious social consequences of such prolonged unemployment as we have had, but it seems that the total effect of the various ameliorative measures at present in operation is still such that a

great residue of persons is left for whom – unless again further measures can be devised – either unemployment insurance or Poor Law relief must be made available for a considerable period.'

55 C. Braithwaite, 'Statistics of finance', in Mess et al., op. cit., p. 203.
56 PRO MH 79/304, *Interim Report of the Lord Mayors' Fund for the Relief of Women and Children in Distressed Mining Areas*, p. 31.
57 See B. Harris, 'Unemployment, insurance and health in interwar Britain', in B. Eichengreen and T. Hatton (eds) *Interwar Unemployment in International Perspective*, Dordrecht, 1988, pp. 149–83.
58 See Harris, 'Medical inspection and the nutrition of schoolchildren in Britain, 1900–1950', pp. 173–248.

13

THE ACHES OF INDUSTRY
Philanthropy and rheumatism in inter-war Britain

David Cantor

It is now commonplace to note that social relationships structured
by gift-exchange are among the most powerful forces which bind a
social group together.[1] Gifts and counter-gifts comprise significant
instruments of social organization, of power, of bonds of kinship,
and of relationships in law. So too, relationships in medicine have
been structured by gift-giving, particularly in the context of medical
philanthropy. Although historians have analysed twentieth-century
British medicine's relations with charity, they have predominantly
focused on individual charities as centres of scientific and medical
research and practice, rather than characterizing the more general
gift-relations structuring medicine.[2] By emphasizing scientific en-
deavours, they overlook some of the comparisons which can be
made with earlier centuries, some of the continuities in gift-giving
and medicine. As yet we know little about the interconnections
between doctors and donors, what impact charity had on medicine
and on the medical profession, what social bonds charity and
gift-giving generated among doctors, why donors gave to medical
charity, and what they expected in return.

Particularly neglected have been the ways in which medical
charities served as links between capital and labour, rich and poor:
symbols of national and imperial unity, undermining expressions of
class or occupational identity. In the rush to describe medicine's
onward and upward progress, too often historians neglect its
relations to social and political struggle, losing sight of the connections between medical and social power. This chapter explores such
connections, suggesting that philanthropy provided an important

site where links between such forms of power were created and recreated. Not that it was the only such site. As Karl Figlio has suggested (following Foucault) power can be diffused through innumerable focuses, obscuring the common-sense notion of actor and acted upon, oppressor and oppressed, ruler and ruled.[3] And this chapter is limited in that it does not venture far from the connections between doctor and donor to explore other sites (such as the doctor–patient relationship) where links between medical and social power were forged. My objective is to analyse the social meanings of philanthropy for doctors and donors, and to illuminate the significance of philanthropy to an understanding of the nature of medical power in inter-war Britain.

Major surveys of British philanthropy during this period tend to downplay the ways in which philanthropy mediates social power. In the most recent account, Frank Prochaska berates studies which treat philanthropy solely as social control, pointing out that the bulk of giving was by the working class for the working class.[4] Social control models may underemphasize the various neighbourly, religious, family and humanitarian ideals that Prochaska identifies among working-class philanthropists. And such models may ignore the ways in which charities have been appropriated by the poor and relatively powerless for their own purposes.[5] Yet Prochaska's account itself downplays the fears and concerns that motivated the founders of some of the more prominent charities. As Gareth Stedman Jones has argued, in the 1860s fears that uncontrolled giving might stimulate social unrest informed the creation of the Charity Organization Society (COS).[6] As J. W. Mason has suggested, by the 1880s such fears were joined by concerns about the emergent socialist movement.[7] Finally, as Joseph Melling and others have argued, philanthropic businessmen established industrial welfare schemes in part in response to work-place conflict, to control local labour markets, maintain managerial prerogative and ameliorate work-place disaffection. As one of Melling's businessmen put it, 'there is no need for us to appear as philanthropists first and business men afterwards – we benefit the workmen incidentally but our motives are selfish to begin with'.[8]

It seems curious then that medical historians have generally assumed that the major medical research charities of the early twentieth century – such as the Imperial Cancer Research Fund (1902), the British Empire Cancer Campaign (1923), the Asthma Research Council (1928) and the Empire Rheumatism Council

(1936) – were immune to such influences. Such neglect is all the more surprising given that historians of campaigning voluntary organizations concerned with, for example, eugenics, social hygiene and family allowances have explored fears of class and national survival among the supporters of such bodies.[9] Many medical members of such organizations were also members of the research charities, as were the businessmen who introduced welfare schemes into their companies.

Put simply my argument is that doctors turned to philanthropy at least in part because they lacked an autonomous source of professional authority and power. When faced with patients with cancer, rheumatism or asthma, these doctors often experienced an unsettling degree of powerlessness in their inability to cure the illness, or to control the patient through long and uncertain courses of treatment. Such experiences, combined with professional and institutional insecurities, prompted medical practitioners to turn to groups outside medicine to make up for their own perceived lack of authority or power. Although this argument grossly oversimplifies a complex and shifting picture of medical attitudes towards philanthropy, such concerns were expressed by doctors themselves. Such a perspective begins to link the creation of medical charities to specific historical events, treating them as creations of their patrons and donors as much as their medical founders.

This chapter is a case study of one of these charities, the Empire Rheumatism Council (ERC), set up in 1936 to unite the growing number of disparate rheumatism organizations established since the First World War.[10] The first such organizations, clinics to treat acute rheumatism and rheumatic heart disease, were products of anxiety about high mortality and disability from heart disease, especially among recruits during the First World War and later among the industrial work-force. By the late 1920s such clinics had been joined by others more concerned with chronic rheumatism (though most saw both acute and chronic conditions). Often these were physical treatment or orthopaedic centres, results of worries about the costs of rheumatism to industry and to the 1911 National Health Insurance scheme. Indeed, such was the momentum, that in 1928–9 these clinics combined with the mineral water hospitals to launch a National Campaign Against Rheumatism. This campaign disappeared in the economic depression of 1929–32, only to be revived as the Empire Rheumatism Council in 1935–6.

The ERC was thus a response to fears that go back to the

nineteenth century of Britain's declining industrial and military position, which were given added impetus by the economic turmoil of the 1920s and early 1930s. As is well known, it was the poor health of British recruits during the Boer War that firmly wedded health to concerns about national efficiency. It was the incidence of heart disease in soldiers during the First World War that performed a similar function for rheumatism, while recession in the early 1920s focused attention on the costs of rheumatic disease to industrial efficiency.[11] But interest in rheumatism was not just about the impact of health on industrial and military inefficiency – it was also about stopping the escalating costs of the National Health Insurance scheme, and about stemming the creeping tide towards state welfare and socialism, and the growing wave of industrial unrest in the 1920s.[12] All these issues came to a head in the crisis of 1929–32 which provided the immediate context for the creation of the council, prompting physicians interested in rheumatism to argue that their specialist skill would help in the revival of the economy, much as orthopaedists and medical hydrologists claimed for their specialities.[13] Finally, as war between Britain and Germany loomed in the late 1930s, the ERC became a symbol of national and imperial unity. Doctors played on all these concerns in their appeals for funds. But the reasons why they did so had as much to do with their own professional insecurities as with these wider issues, and it is with the doctors' insecurities that I begin.

To many doctors the creation of the ERC was as unsettling as it was welcome. While it promised to focus the nation's generosity on rheumatism, it also heightened many institutional, epistemological and technical uncertainties as doctors fought each other for what they saw as a limited pool of funds. Side by side on the ERC sat clinicians and clinical and laboratory scientists, advocates of physical medicine and advocates of vaccine therapy, practitioners from the mineral water hospitals and from town clinics, from London and from the provinces. In the preceding years many of these groups had been at loggerheads with each other, and while the creation of the council symbolized their unity, it also heightened their competition. For example each of the three major English mineral water hospitals launched their own national appeals in 1937–8, ostensibly as a part of the ERC's united campaign, but also as a means of protecting themselves from long-standing competition from each other and from burgeoning urban rheumatism clinics.[14] In turn, these urban clinics began their own appeals. Thus in London, the Charterhouse

Rheumatism Clinic (CRC) launched its own national appeal in 1937–8,[15] an appeal that was of particular concern to what was the most prominent clinic of its day, the rheumatism clinic at Peto Place in London. As I shall indicate, the CRC's emphasis on vaccine therapy was anathema to many of the physicians at Peto Place.

In 1937–8 the CRC's appeal appeared as a major threat to the future of Peto Place, both reducing the chances of it launching a successful appeal of its own, and undermining the ERC. The physicians at Peto Place had seen the ERC as offering salvation from the financial difficulties that had plagued it since 1929 when the Red Cross founded it as the centre-piece of the National Campaign Against Rheumatism.[16]

The competition between clinics was complicated by debates over the shape of medical specialization. With the exception of the Charterhouse Rheumatism Clinic, most clinics adopted physical techniques as the mainstay of treatment. Yet there was no agreement whether physicians using such techniques should be classified as specialists in disease or technique. Some physicians in rheumatism clinics in the spa towns felt that being classified as technique specialists undermined their ability to compete with clinics in industrial and large urban centres. Thus the physician at the rheumatism clinic in the spa town of Droitwich, J. W. T. Patterson, claimed that the spas were losing their leadership in the treatment of rheumatism because spa physicians preferred to specialize not in the rheumatic diseases, but in techniques.[17] His opponents argued the opposite point, namely that specialization in 'spa practice' was necessary to protect the spas from the competition of London physicians. To them, the spas could not hope to compete for out-patients with clinics based in major urban and industrial areas on the doorsteps of sick and disabled people.[18]

By 1935 the latter had persuaded the International Society for Medical Hydrology that spa practitioners should be treated only as specialists in technique.[19] To those who agreed with Patterson, this move could have barred spa clinics from playing a significant role in the ERC's campaign, for, inevitably, when someone proposed specializing in technique, it raised questions about the technical specialists' skill in dealing with the disease they treated. Such an eventuality could have had severe repercussions for the medical economy of the spa town. As the town clerk of Leamington put it, a rheumatism clinic 'would undoubtedly mean a big increase in the importance of Leamington as a Spa and also in the numbers of people visiting the town in search of health'.[20]

Battles for funding also reveal the ways in which medical authority could depend on donors, as the case of H. Warren Crowe, the founder of the Charterhouse Rheumatism Clinic, illustrates.[21] Crowe, a student of the pioneer of vaccine therapy, Almroth Wright, believed that all rheumatic diseases were bacterial in origin and amenable to vaccine therapy; he had founded the CRC in 1928 to provide vaccine treatment for rheumatic patients.[22] Such a position was anathema to the founders of the ERC, who, while they could not dismiss vaccine therapy out of hand, emphasized instead the primacy of physical methods.[23] Many founders felt that Crowe himself was little more than a quack, and his staff barely competent in the treatment of rheumatic disease, and as a consequence it is hardly surprising that Crowe was not a member of the ERC when it was formed.[24] Nevertheless, his scheme was at least as successful as that of the Red Cross. By 1933 a new clinic had been opened in Hallam Street, but even that proved too small, and (as we have seen) in 1937–8 Crowe launched his own national appeal on the back of the ERC's. His critics commented in frustration at Crowe's ability to charm support out of people.

'What a nuisance this fellow is!' wrote Lord Horder, chairman of the council, to the secretary of the ERC after Crowe had launched his national appeal against rheumatism, 'He has influential backing, as of course you know.'[25] Indeed, in some cases Crowe seemed to be having more success in attracting donors than the ERC: for example he secured £5,000 in 1938 from Lord Nuffield, who had anonymously given only £50 to the ERC in 1935.[26] Perhaps in response to their own fund-raising difficulties, in 1937–8 the ERC offered Crowe a place on its council. Crowe accepted this position while continuing to poach what the ERC regarded as its donors.[27] In 1938 he secured perhaps his ultimate coup, when he engaged the Duchess of Gloucester, the wife of the patron of the ERC, to open a new centre-piece clinic in Weymouth Street, financed by his 1937–8 appeal.[28]

Similarly disputes between laboratory scientists and clinicians for authority on health matters were also shaped by donors.[29] In 1936 Edward Mellanby, the secretary of the Medical Research Council, the bastion of laboratory research, upset Horder by telling him that it was nonsense to appeal for research money, as the MRC would give £1,000 a year immediately if they found anyone with a really bright idea in the field who was prepared and competent to work it out.[30] The MRC itself claimed it had little idea as to what clues to follow in researching rheumatism. Nevertheless, once it looked like the appeal was going to be a success, Mellanby was eager enough to accept an MRC-appointed majority on the ERC's Scientific Advisory Committee. Both Mellanby and his predecessor, Walter Fletcher, feared the ability of the clinicians to play on their personal contacts with patients. In defining medical science, clinicians thus had an unfair advantage over laboratory scientists who, Mellanby and Fletcher felt, did not have similar power. Fletcher stated:

> It does not have to be fought so much in other countries, but in England, the Court and the Ministries and the newspaper proprietors are apt to get their ideas of medical science from the successful practitioner with whom they come in personal contact, and to whom they may feel indebted for personal services.[31]

Fletcher was thus suspicious of, if not at times downright hostile to, clinician involvement in raising funds for medical research fearing that it would perpetuate their control over laboratory research.

Many of the donors and lay members of the ERC were personal friends and family of its medical founders, and membership of other voluntary organizations stretched these personal networks further. Such networks of family, friendship and acquaintance are notoriously difficult to reconstruct, even in this case where only a dozen or so people provided over 80 per cent of the ERC's pre-war income, and one donor, Alexander Maclean, the eponymous founder of the toothpaste company, provided £13,000, about 29 per cent of the total.[32] Nevertheless, the ERC's files suggest that the key figures were a small group of London-based physicians with strong links with Peto Place and the British Empire Cancer Campaign on which the ERC was partly modelled.[33]

Of these physicians the most prominent was probably Lord Horder, a royal physician, and chairman of the council. As Greta Jones has pointed out, Horder's interests in health and social matters were wide ranging. He was President of the Eugenics Society, a member of the Institute of Management, and involved in smoke and noise abatement, mental hygiene, family planning, the Boy Scouts, the General Council for Physical Recreations and the provision of National Parks.[34] In addition he was a founder member of the British Empire Cancer Campaign (BECC), a defender of the voluntary hospital system and an advocate of greater hospital provision for middle-class patients.[35] Horder shared the platform defending the voluntary hospital system in public speeches with a number of other patrons and donors to the ERC.[36] In addition his fund-raising and social activities ensured that he circulated among the circles of the men and women who supported the campaign. For example he attended a meeting with the Member of Parliament (MP), H. P. Croft, and Alexander Maclean (both patrons of ERC) to celebrate the latter's donation to the Royal Victoria and West Hants Hospital and Eventide Homes in Bournemouth,[37] and a meeting of the London Hampshire Society with his friend and patient, the retailer, John Spedan Lewis.[38] Among his personal friends Horder counted other patrons of the council, the Conservative MP, John Gretton (who donated £960 18s. 2d.), and the GEC (General Electric Company) industrialist, Hugo Hirst (£25).[39] Indeed at one time he complained to his right-hand man, the Peto Place physician, W. S. C. Copeman, that the latter was relying only on Horder's friends to launch the rheumatism appeal.[40] For his part, Copeman secured support from his family and in-laws – his wife gave £105, his mother-in-law £205, his father £100, his mother also £100 and he gave £235 personally.[41] The Red Cross, with which both Horder, Copeman and another founding physician, William Willcox, already had contacts through Peto Place and the BECC, donated £1,001.

These three physicians – Horder, Willcox and Copeman, the chairman, vice-chairman and medical secretary respectively – seem to have been the key medical figures in launching the ERC successfully. Nevertheless, other physicians also raised significant funds. The Scottish physician, L. S. P. Davidson, secured £1,100 from an anonymous donor, and provided Frank Fox, the lay secretary of the council, with letters of introduction to another patron, the Unionist MP, Sir Robert Horne.[42] They all attended various fund-raising events, and spoke at public meetings on behalf of the campaign. In these activities they were joined by a number of others such as the Medical Officer of Health, James Fenton, the Manipulative Surgeon to the King, Sir Morton Smart, and the Lister Institute scientist, Lady Ruth Balfour, who spoke at numerous public meetings between 1936 and 1939 to publicize the council's campaign.[43]

Yet doctors were not alone in pushing for a rheumatism campaign. The Leeds-fund-raiser, B. T. Clegg, almost single-handedly ran his own rheumatism campaign in the north of England before the ERC was formed. He argued that disease and social campaigns were a useful way of popularizing university-based laboratory research, and stated that 'as a pure business proposition, the best way to decrease the need for hospital treatment is to increase medical research'.[44] His major concern was that the rheumatism appeal should not develop into the provision of baths and other 'doubtful' treatments, and Clegg seems to have been an influential adviser to Horder and Copeman on the appeal in the north and the establishment of the ERC.[45] Similarly Copeman was confident enough of the support of Spedan Lewis to suggest that he and some others might be encouraged 'to decentralise and virtually run little "corners" of the campaign'.[46]

Appeals targeted a number of groups, but predominantly approved societies and industry. To the former the ERC pointed out that between one-sixth and one-seventh of the total sickness benefits went on diseases classed as rheumatic, and cost the National Health Insurance scheme £1,840,000 a year in sickness benefit.[47] It is a measure of the success of this appeal that the Prudential Approved Society was the second largest donor to the ERC before the Second World War, contributing £5,000. In the case of industry, the founders of the ERC aimed to attract interest from what they termed 'public men of influence' who were also 'enlightened employers of labour'.[48] Appeals to these 'enlightened' people touched on concerns about the effect of rheumatism on efficiency. 'It goes without saying that you are aware of the vast and largely preventable ravages which this group of diseases makes into the hours and efficiency of labour annually,'[49] noted the letter of appeal to industrialists. And much publicity stressed the statistic that 3,141,000 weeks of work were lost annually by the insured population alone, a figure first highlighted by a 1924 Ministry of Health report. This may explain the fact that 56 per cent of donors in 1936 ran businesses.[50]

The ERC founders also tried to canvass political support from both the Labour movement and from the Conservative Party. In the event mainly Conservative and Unionist MPs joined the council – H. P. Croft, John Gretton, Harold Sutcliffe – along with the independent medical MP, E. Graham-Little and the national Labour MP, Sidney Markham. The Labour movement was represented by the President of the TUC, Ernest Bevin, who had recently retired from membership of the MRC's Industrial Health Research Board.

Finally, the doctors also appealed to women – Lady Rhondda (editor of *Time and Tide*), Lady Aberdeen and Temair (President of the People's League of Health and founder of the Women's National

Association in 1907) and Lady Ruth Balfour (Vice-President of the National Council of Women) being the notable figures. Indeed B. T. Clegg categorized rheumatism as a disease that would particularly appeal to women:

> The Cancer Campaign has been a man's job, a Rheumatism Campaign would be a woman's job, the Nerve and Mental Diseases Campaign would be a man's job, and the Children's Diseases Campaign would be a woman's job.[51]

Lady Balfour argued that the National Council of Women and other women's organizations should see that provision was made for detecting acute and sub-acute rheumatism in children in order to combat heart disease. 'Then, if in any area they could establish a clinic for chronic rheumatism . . . they would be doing a tremendous thing, and justifying their position as a society.'[52]

None of the donors and patrons to the ERC gave reasons for joining the ERC. Some, such as the Bournemouth MP, H. P. Croft, and his wife had rheumatism, while experiences of ill-health may have motivated others, such as the MP, Harold Sutcliffe.[53] But personal experiences of illness were not the only interests that donors and patrons had in common. Many were involved in voluntary activities such as the BECC, the Royal Bath Hospital at Harrogate,[54] the St John Clinic and Institute of Physical Medicine,[55] the Chamberlain Centenary Fund,[56] a 1936 recruitment campaign for the Territorial Army,[57] the Queen's Hospital for Children in Hackney,[58] the National Advertisement Benevolent Fund,[59] and 'Old Ben', the newsvendors' charity.[60] A number saw voluntarism as a defence against the encroachment of the state. For example Lord Iliffe, speaking as President of the Queen's Hospital for Children in Hackney, noted that despite the huge financial problems faced by the voluntary hospitals, he felt that it was essential that they be retained at all costs. The voluntary system, he felt, was more elastic, more sympathetic and more human than institutions run by the state or by municipalities.[61] Horder, whose support for voluntarism has already been noted, went even further, suggesting that business enterprise was almost a form of voluntarism. Both activities relied on an individualist ethic, and were necessary defences against the state. Thus he told the Annual Conference of the British Commercial Gas Association:

> A good many things which in other countries are left to

a central bureau are done here by the people themselves
as a result of their own initiative. And they are sometimes
done very well. You are, I believe, examples of successful
business concerns which combine public benefits with private
enterprise.[62]

Such claims would have gone down well with the Gas Light and
Coke Company, which had already given £200 to the ERC.

A number of donors and patrons saw commercial opportunities
in the ERC. An advertisement for the 'Lancelot' gas-fire appeared in
the ERC's academic journal, the *Annals of the Rheumatic Diseases*,
suggesting that such fires were an effective component of therapy
for rheumatic conditions.[63] Many commercial spas also tried to
capitalize on the ERC's campaign, offering themselves as centres
for the treatment of rheumatism.[64] To retailers such as Selfridge
and Spedan Lewis philanthropy was also probably part of the
gimmickry of salesmanship. In 1932 the latter appointed a Director
of Goodwill at his store in Oxford Street to deal with customer
complaints and to make charitable donations. 'In the ordinary
way there is a staff committee to deal with donations,' noted
Mr Watkins, newly appointed to the post,[65] 'but there are, of
course, gifts which have business motives, and these are made by
the goodwill director.' Charity and health also blurred easily into
advertising when exhibitions were held in the various stores. At the
time the ERC was formed, Lewis combined with Selfridge and other
London traders in an annual Christmas appeal collecting dolls and
toys for sick children, which was aimed at shoppers in their stores.[66]
Also in 1935, Selfridge organized a health and housing exhibition in
his store in Oxford Street, while later in the year, as part of the Bread
Publicity Campaign, his store-front had the sign 'Selfridge's Bread
the Key to Health and Vigour'.[67]

Related to the concern about the encroaching state was a fear
of socialism. Many of the donors and patrons to the ERC were
anti-socialist, including Spedan Lewis, Lord Iliffe, Gordon Selfridge,
Lord Hirst, Lord Nuffield, Graham-Little and, of course, the
Conservative MPs, Croft, Gretton and Sutcliffe. Lord Iliffe thought
that the only problem with capitalism was that capital was in
too few hands. He argued that by creating more capitalists, not
only would capitalism be cured of its ills, but also Bolshevism
would be destroyed.[68] His views would have been shared by
the advocates of profit-sharing such as the Prudential Assurance

Company (represented by Joseph Burn), Lord Leverhulme and John Spedan Lewis, all of whom had introduced profit-sharing schemes in response to industrial unrest and socialism.[69] As Lewis put it, '[p]artnership is the only hope of preventing the rank and file of the Great Western democracies from embarking on premature socialistic experiments'.[70]

For Lewis such schemes might help to stem British decline. In his view not only might they turn the work-force into capitalists, but also the schemes demanded an ethic of service, perhaps even sacrifice, from owners who had to forgo the comfort of entering public service with their capital safely invested. Using himself as an example, he explained that businessmen had to remain at the helm of their businesses, rather than retire and enter Parliament.[71] Charity also served a similar function, and demanded similar service. Lord Croft, for example, commented on Alexander Maclean's gift to Bournemouth that 'Britain will never decline so long as her sons realise that the privileges of citizenship and power call also for the response of service'.[72]

Other employers connected with the ERC were also interested in bridging the gap between the two sides of industry, especially after the heated industrial unrest of the 1920s. An example is Hugo Hirst, a participant in the Mond–Turner talks inaugurated in 1927 after the failure of the General Strike the previous year. These talks were started by Alfred Mond (the founder of ICI) in the hope of ushering in a period of industrial peace by setting up joint negotiating bodies between unions and employers. Mond himself was anti-socialist, and believed that the best defence against socialism was a happy, contented and industrious work-force.[73] There is little to suggest that Hirst felt otherwise, and one Labour politician later noted that Hirst worked like a 'Trojan' to bring capital and labour together during these talks.[74] Indeed, the ERC seemed to underscore the rapprochement between capital and labour set in motion by the Mond–Turner talks, for two participants in those talks were lay members of council – Hirst for the employers and Ernest Bevin for the unions. Ernest Bevin, in 1936 the President of the TUC, had joined the Mond–Turner talks against some opposition from within the trade union movement. In response to criticism Bevin argued the case for collaboration with management so that the work-force would have a say in issues such as rationalization, which had important ramifications for workers, but which employers in the past had been unwilling to talk over with unions. The ERC also stressed the common interest of employers and employees, this time in combating rheumatism.[75]

Yet, if charity symbolized the unity and common purpose between workers and employers, it also highlighted those who opposed such unity. For Spedan Lewis, both management and labour were bound together by his partnership, and had common interests against both the fermenters of industrial disruption and the financial sharks of the City. A certain loyalty was therefore expected of the work-force, a point brought home by Mr Ivan Snell, a Marylebone magistrate, to one employee caught stealing from Spedan Lewis's Oxford Street store. In fining this employee Mr Snell commented that the defendant actually deserved hard labour and prison for stealing from what 'was practically a *charitable* organisation of the best description for the benefit of their employees'.[76] And it was not a far step to extend such rationales from individual charities and businesses to the nation itself. While on the one hand Spedan Lewis hoped that his partnership schemes would save western democracy, on the other hand, Selfridge returned from the United States of America in 1932 to declare that democracy was a failure, and that in 100 or 200 years no democracies would exist. As one paper quoted Selfridge's judgement, 'what must eventually come is the control of a country by an inspiring, unselfish spirit, managing it as a great business is managed'.[77]

Finally, some of the donors and patrons to the Empire Rheumatism Council had imperial interests – at least five patrons and donors helped launch a Campaign for Imperial Co-operation in 1936 through the Joseph Chamberlain Centenary Fund, to strengthen the economic and military bonds within the Empire.[78] The chairman of this group was the Bournemouth MP, H. P. Croft,[79] an anti-free-trader who favoured imperial preference and was a one-time stalwart of Joseph Chamberlain's tariff reform crusade. His activities in the later 1930s were dominated by German demands for the return of the colonies taken from them after the First World War to which he was adamantly opposed.[80] 'The first fact to grasp', he wrote in 1938, 'is that the Mandated Territories are not ours to hand out like so many charitable gifts.'[81] The Empire was, for him, a bulwark of democracy, a defence against Germany and against communism and he bitterly criticized socialists for wanting to break it up. These German demands prompted Croft to contrast what he felt was the German conception of Empire with the more benevolent one of the British. In his view, Germany exploited her colonies at the expense of indigenous peoples, while the British sought to raise each colony up step-by-step eventually to equal status with the mother country. Clearly the creation of the ERC in 1936, and its efforts to stimulate similar ventures in New Zealand, Australia and Canada, can have done little harm to Croft's portrayal of Empire. Newspapers depicted the Dominions rallying to the Campaign, with London as their centre, a theme of imperial unity that became increasingly important as war with Germany seemed likely.[82] Then, in the last years of the decade, the metaphors of war that had characterized the rheumatism campaigns of the 1920s and 1930s were given added power by the prospect of real hostilities.[83] To Spedan Lewis and Graham-Little the rheumatism campaign offered practical advantages in improved health in the coming fight.[84] To the Duke of Gloucester the ERC was symbolic of British resolve and unity in the face of German threats.[85]

To many donors charities served to cement the bonds of society, uniting capital and labour, Britain and her Empire, even unifying the nation in the face of Nazi Germany and stemming British decline. As Croft implied in his discussion of German imperial demands, charity was a symbol of power and property, a means of combating socialism, industrial unrest and creeping state welfare, of reproducing specific social structures – welfare rather than confrontational capitalism. While donors and patrons may have emphasized consensus rather than confrontation, partnership rather than exploitation, charity was also defined by certain power relations. It was in many ways the benevolent means by which elites tried to maintain social order, and where charity failed the full weight of the law could come down. Hence anyone who abused a 'charity' was challenging not only the people whom it was intended to benefit, but also the means by which the powerful maintained their authority, as the man who stole from the John Lewis Partnership found out to his cost.

But to what extent did the charities' reassertion of the links between employers and employees, the bonds of deference and obligation which philanthropists attempted to create undermine class consciousness, working-class solidarity? There is as yet no answer, for we know little about working-class attitudes towards the council. The ERC itself gained little financial support from working-class donors, though certain clinics and hospitals attracted substantial working-class support. Further work is needed to address how clinics and hospitals in their interactions with patients embodied the class relations of their creators – and how such interests were perceived and acted upon by patients. Despite the interest in 'the patient' among historians of earlier centuries, few historians of twentieth-century medicine have begun to integrate patients into their analyses. A full account of philanthropy will be achieved only with such an integration.

If we cannot be certain of the effects of charity on class consciousness, we do know that doctors perceived their interests in alignment with philanthropy. They may have worried about the extent to which commercial pressures polluted medicine.[86] But in the competition for funds, doctors inevitably sided with richer donors, at least in the ERC, and regularly played on their concerns – not only the cost of the National Health Insurance scheme, but also worries about efficiency, unemployment, rationalization, industrial unrest, socialism and the future of the Empire. Such competition ensured that donors not only provided the rheumatism centres, but also shaped, in part, pre-war 'rheumatology', forcing otherwise hostile doctors together. Although the founders of the ERC might refuse to collaborate scientifically with Warren Crowe, once they were faced with donors who were willing to accord Crowe equivalent scientific credibility, they had little option but to co-opt him in fighting rheumatism. Such 'shot-gun weddings' illuminate medicine's lack of an autonomous professional power base, highlight the ways in which the professional structure of medicine was shaped by outside interests, and suggest that at times the authority of medical science was little more than a by-product of wider struggles over social stability and national survival.

NOTES

The ERC's records are now held by the Arthritis and Rheumatism Council for Research (ARC). They are not catalogued in a systematic fashion, and consequently I have referenced files by their name. Other records come from the *Daily Telegraph*'s cuttings collection. It is not always clear which publications the cuttings are taken from. Consequently these records are referenced according to the subject of the particular collection and the date of cutting – for example 'DT (Iliffe), 2 May 1932' refers to a cutting for that date in Lord Iliffe's folder. Other archives are the Medical Research Council (MRC) and the Public Record Office (Kew) (PRO). Aside from the *Daily Telegraph*, cuttings come predominantly from the cuttings' books of the ARC, the John Lewis Partnership archives, Selfridge's archives, the Sutcliffe papers (held by his son, J. H. V. Sutcliffe) and the Croft papers held at Churchill College, Cambridge.

1 The classic formulation is M. Mauss, *The Gift: Forms and Functions of Exchange in Archaic Societies*, London, 1954.
2 J. Austoker, *A History of the Imperial Cancer Research Fund, 1902–1986*, Oxford, 1988; A. R. Hall and B. A. Bembridge, *Physic and Philanthropy: A History of the Wellcome Trust, 1936–1986*, Cambridge, 1986; L. Granshaw, *St Mark's Hospital: A Social History of a Specialist Hospital*, London, 1985; J. Beinart, *A History of the Nuffield Department of Anaesthetics, Oxford, 1937–1987*, Oxford, 1987. See also R. Clark, *A Biography of the Nuffield Foundation*, London, 1972. For comparison see S. Cavallo, 'Charity, power, and patronage in eighteenth-century Italian hospitals: the case of Turin', in L. Granshaw and R. Porter (eds) *The Hospital in History*, London and New York, 1989; R. Porter, 'The gift relation: philanthropy and provincial hospitals in eighteenth-century England', in ibid., pp. 149–78.
3 K. Figlio, 'How does illness mediate social relations? Workmen's compensation and medico-legal practices, 1890–1940', in P. Wright and A. Treacher (eds) *The Problem of Medical Knowledge: Examining the Social Construction of Medicine*, Edinburgh, 1982.
4 F. Prochaska, *The Voluntary Impulse: Philanthropy in Modern Britain*, London and Boston, Mass., 1988.
5 F. M. L. Thomson, 'Social control in Victorian Britain', *Economic History Review*, 1981, vol. 34; G. Stedman Jones, 'Class expression versus social control? A critique of recent trends in the history of "leisure"', *Languages of Class: Studies in Working Class History 1832–1982*, Cambridge, 1983.
6 G. Stedman Jones, *Outcast London: A Study in the Relationship Between Classes in Victorian Society*, Oxford, 1971, ch. 13. The standard account of COS is C. L. Mowat, *The Charity Organisation Society, 1869–1913*, London, 1961.
7 J. W. Mason, 'Thomas Mackay: the anti-socialist philosophy of the Charity Organisation Society', in K. D. Brown (ed.) *Essays in Anti-Labour History: Responses to the Rise of Labour in Britain*, London and Basingstoke, 1974.
8 J. Melling, 'Employers, industrial welfare, and the struggle for workplace control in British industry', in H. F. Gospel and C. R. Littler (eds) *Managerial Strategies and Industrial Relations: An Historical and Comparative Study*, London, 1983, quotation at p. 62; Melling, 'Employers, industrial housing, and the evolution of company welfare policies in Britain's heavy industry: West Scotland, 1870–1920', *International Review of Social History*, 1981, vol. 26; Melling, 'Industrial strife and business welfare philosophy: the case of the South Metropolitan Gas Company from the 1880s to the War', *Business History*, 1979, vol. 21; R. Fitzgerald, *British Labour Management and Industrial Welfare 1846–1939*, London, 1988; H. Jones, 'Employers' welfare schemes and industrial relations in inter-war Britain', *Business History*, 1983, vol. 25. See also N. Whiteside, 'Industrial welfare and labour regulation in Britain at the time of the First World War', *International Review of Social History*, 1980, vol. 25.

9 The literature on this field is voluminous, but see D. Kevles, *In the Name of Eugenics*, New York, 1985; G. R. Searle, *Eugenics and Politics in Britain 1900–1914*, Leyden, 1976; D. Mackenzie, 'Sociobiologies in competition: the Biometrician–Mendelian Debate', in C. Webster (ed.) *Biology, Medicine and Society, 1840–1940*, Cambridge, 1981; M. Freeden, 'Eugenics and progressive thought: a study in ideological affinity', *Historical Journal*, 1979, vol. 22; G. Jones, 'Eugenics and social policy between the wars', *Historical Journal*, 1982, vol. 25; G. Jones, *Social Hygiene in Twentieth Century Britain*, London, 1986; J. Macnicol, *The Movement for Family Allowances*, London, 1981.

10 D. Cantor, *These Rheumatic Isles: A Social History of British Rheumatism Charities, 1920–1986*, forthcoming.

11 G. R. Searle, *The Quest for National Efficiency*, Oxford, 1971; J. Howell, '"Soldier's Heart": the redefinition of heart disease and speciality formation in twentieth-century Great Britain', *Medical History Supplement*, 1985, no. 5; Cantor, op. cit.

12 N. Whiteside, 'Counting the cost: sickness and disability among working people in an era of industrial recession, 1920–39', *Economic History Review*, 1987, vol. 40.

13 R. Cooter, *Surgery and Society in Peace and War: The Making of Modern Orthopaedics, 1880–1945*, forthcoming; D. Cantor, 'The contradictions of specialisation: rheumatism and the decline of the spa in inter-war Britain', *Medical History Supplement*, 1990, no. 10.

14 Cantor, forthcoming, op. cit.; see also Cantor, 1990, op. cit. For details of the appeals of the three major spa hospitals see 'Great Bath appeal . . .', *Bath and Wilts Chronicle*, 28 January 1937; 'Devonshire Royal Hospital', *Buxton Advertiser*, 7 August 1937; 'Hospital that is solvent', *Leeds Mercury*, 27 February 1937.

15 'Lord Nuffield's £5000 for clinic', *The Times*, 6 August 1938.

16 For details of the problems of Peto Place see Cantor, forthcoming, op. cit.

17 J. W. T. Patterson, 'The British spas and the problem of rheumatism – the need for organisation and authority', *Archives of Medical Hydrology*, 1932, vol. 10, p. 100.

18 A. P. Cawadias, 'The health resort physician', *Archives of Medical Hydrology*, 1932, vol. 10, pp. 98–9.

19 'Medical ethics for spa practitioners', *Archives of Medical Hydrology*, 1935, vol. 13, p. 51.

20 'Proposed rheumatic clinic', *Leamington Chronicle*, 12 November 1937.

21 Crowe wrote his own account of the history of the Charterhouse Rheumatism Clinic, 'The Charterhouse Rheumatism Clinic'. I am grateful to Virginia Crowe for providing me with a copy of this and other documentation.

22 H. Warren Crowe, *Handbook of the Vaccine Treatment of Chronic Rheumatic Diseases*, 3rd edn, London and Oxford, 1939.

23 See for example the comments in the textbooks by the following members of the ERC. W. S. C. Copeman, *The Treatment of Rheumatism in General Practice*, 2nd edn, London, 1935; F. G. Thomson and

R. G. Gordon, *Chronic Rheumatic Diseases: Their Diagnosis and Treatment*, London and Oxford, 1926; F. J. Poynton and B. Schlesinger, *Recent Advances in the Study of Rheumatism*, 2nd edn, London, 1937. For a less partisan treatment of Crowe's vaccine therapy from an advocate of physical methods see G. D. Kersley, *The Rheumatic Diseases: A Concise Manual for the Practitioner*, London, 1934.

24 See for example the comments on Dr Ogg by L. S. P. Davidson to Lord Horder, 10 October 1945, ARC archives: 'Charterhouse Rheumatism Clinic'.

25 Lord Horder to F. Fox, 26 August 1938, ARC archives: 'Charterhouse Rheumatism Clinic'. For similar comments see L. J. Witts to F. G. C. Herrald, 26 April 1940, MRC:1063/14.

26 *The Times*, 6 August 1938, op. cit. Nuffield's gift is not recorded in the annual reports, but is mentioned by B. T. Clegg in a letter to Frank Fox, 30 November 1935, ARC archives: 'Organisation and Minutes of R.C.P. Committee on Rheumatic Diseases'. Also the Charterhouse Rheumatism Clinic approached Mrs Gretton, wife of the Rt Hon. John Gretton MP, asking for support. Lady St John of Bletso to Mrs Gretton, 26 July 1937, ARC archives: 'Charterhouse Rheumatism Clinic'.

27 For example Crowe tried to tempt the John Lewis Partnership into his fold in 1939. T. W. Robinson (Director of the John Lewis Partnership) to A. R. Peers (Charterhouse Clinic), 28 April 1939, and T. W. Robinson to F. Fox, 28 September 1939, ARC archives: 'Charterhouse Rheumatism Clinic'.

28 *The Times*, 6 August 1938, op. cit.

29 I am grateful to Daniel Fox for pointing out that the ERC also became a focus of struggles not only between clinicians and laboratory scientists, but also between the latter and clinical scientists.

30 W. S. C. Copeman to F. Fox, 1 February 1937, ARC archives: 'Organisation and minutes of R.C.P. Committee on Rheumatic Diseases'. See also MRC:1063/15.

31 W. Fletcher to W. A. Robinson, 28 July 1923, MRC:1383 vol. 2.

32 Details of the amounts donated by Maclean and others are taken from the annual reports of the ERC and refer to the total given before the outbreak of war.

33 Horder and the vice-chairman of the ERC, William Willcox, shared a common membership in the BECC with ERC patrons such as the MP, E. Graham-Little, the retailer, John Spedan Lewis (who donated £1,000), the Leeds fund-raiser, B. T. Clegg (£50), Captain E. C. Chapman, and the MP, Harold Sutcliffe.

34 G. Jones, 1986, op. cit., p. 56.

35 'Future of voluntary hospitals', *The Times*, 22 June 1928; 'Health resorts conference: Buxton's new clinic', *British Medical Journal*, 4 May 1935, pp. 940–1.

36 E. Graham-Little and Lord Iliffe were also vigorous supporters of the voluntary hospital system. *The Times*, 22 June 1928, 'Hospital's care for children', DT (Iliffe), 2 May 1939. For some doubts about the ability of the voluntary hospital system to cope with rheumatism by another founder of the ERC see L. S. P. Davidson, 'Can the voluntary hospital

system solve the problem of rheumatic disease?', in *Proceedings of the International Congress on Rheumatism and Hydrology (London and Oxford) and the Bicentenary Congress on Chronic Rheumatism (Bath), March 25th to April 2nd 1938*, London, 1938.

37 '£10,000 gift for the hospital', *Bournemouth Daily Echo*, 24 October 1936.

38 Cartoon, 'With the Hampshiremen', *Tatler*, 9 December 1936. I am grateful to the archivist of the John Lewis Partnership, for informing me that Spedan Lewis was Horder's patient.

39 W. S. C. Copeman to F. Fox, 1 February 1937, op. cit.

40 Ibid.

41 I am grateful to W. S. C. Copeman's son, Peter Copeman, for pointing out that his father married the daughter of Mrs W. W. Bourne, of Bournes of Oxford Street. Peter Copeman also suggested that his father was instrumental in getting the donation of James Roberts (£2,800); however, I have been unable to substantiate this.

42 W. S. C. Copeman to F. Fox, 1 February 1937, op. cit.

43 Cantor, forthcoming, op. cit.

44 B. T. Clegg to J. B. Baillie, 28 June 1935. See also B. T. Clegg to J. B. Baillie, 30 May 1930, Leeds University archives: 'General correspondence 1923–1937', G-2 Registry Departmental [CFO-H], Medicine, Box 18, Folder H.24, Rheumatism.

45 On Clegg's involvement in the Northern campaigns see Cantor, forthcoming, op. cit. It was probably Clegg who suggested Frank Fox as secretary to the ERC: B. T. Clegg to W. S. C. Copeman, 16 October 1935; B. T. Clegg to F. Fox, 30 November 1935, ARC archives: 'Organisation and minutes of R.C.P. Committee on Rheumatic Diseases'.

46 W. S. C. Copeman, 'A few "great thoughts" on the E.R.C. for 1937', 3 January 1937; J. Spedan Lewis to Horder, 2 March 1936, ARC archives: 'Organisation and minutes of R.C.P. Committee on Rheumatic Diseases'.

47 These figures were first outlined in Ministry of Health, *Reports on Public Health and Medical Subjects No. 23: The Incidence of Rheumatic Diseases*, London, 1924.

48 Draft letter to Lord Leverhulme, 1 October 1935, ARC archives: 'Organisation and minutes of R.C.P. Committee on Rheumatic Diseases'.

49 Ibid.

50 Ministry of Health, 1924, op. cit.

51 B. T. Clegg to J. B. Baillie, 30 May 1930, op. cit.

52 'Steps to combat rheumatism', *Surrey Advertiser*, 10 June 1937. See also 'Rheumatic diseases in North-East Scotland', *Aberdeen Press and Journal*, 20 May 1937; 'Rheumatism and nutrition', *Middlesex County Times*, 5 June 1937.

53 'The Borough Member: laid up with attack of rheumatism', *Bournemouth Daily Echo*, 28 January 1930; 'The Hon. Lady Croft', *Bournemouth Daily Echo*, 24 December 1937; B. T. Clegg, 'Tribute to Sir Harold Sutcliffe', *Hebden Bridge Times*, 31 January 1958. For a jibe at the self-interest of those with rheumatism supporting an anti-rheumatism dinner see the comments on Cardinal Hinsley and

the Duke of Gloucester in 'Next Please . . .', *Daily Express*, 17 January 1938.

54 The Earl of Harewood, a patron of the ERC, was President of the Royal Bath Hospital.

55 The Earl of Scarbrough, a patron of the ERC, was Chairman of the clinic.

56 Lord Iliffe (newspaper proprietor) met Lord Nuffield (car manufacturer) at the Chamberlain Centenary Fund in 1936: J. Barnes and D. Nicholson, *The Empire at Bay: The Leo Amery Diaries, 1929–1945*, London, 1988, p. 420.

57 Spedan Lewis, Lord Hirst, Gordon Selfridge (Oxford Street retailer), and J. Burn (Prudential Approved Society), along with Lord Austin (motor cars) who had recently given an evasive reply to requests for funds: 'Luncheon', *The Times*, 20 November 1936.

58 Lord Iliffe and Frank Bowater (Lord Mayor of London): 'Hospital's care for children', DT (Iliffe), 2 May 1939.

59 Lord Iliffe and Viscount Leverhulme: '£10,300 subscribed at dinner', DT (Iliffe), 28 April 1934.

60 Sir Francis Goodenough and Lord Iliffe: '"Old Ben's" 95th Dinner', DT (Iliffe), 23 October 1934.

61 'Hospital's care for children', DT (Iliffe), 2 May 1939.

62 Lord Horder, 'Heat, health and happiness', *Gas World*, 29 April 1939, quotation at p. 385.

63 'Gas fires in the treatment of rheumatism', *Annals of the Rheumatic Diseases*, July 1939, vol. 1, pt 3, p. iii.

64 Cantor, forthcoming, op. cit.

65 'Director of goodwill', *Draper's Record*, 14 May 1932.

66 'Buy an extra doll or toy', *Daily Sketch (Manchester Edition)*, 28 November 1936.

67 'Housing and health exhibition', *Municipal Journal*, 15 March 1935; 'Selfridge's health and housing exhibition', *Morning Post*, 19 March 1935. On the bread advertisement see photograph in *P.L.R. Bulletin*, July 1935, p. 72.

68 '£3,000,000,000 held by small investors', DT (Iliffe), 5 June 1935; 'Britain a land of capitalists', DT (Iliffe), 27 September 1937.

69 E. Bristow, 'Profit-sharing, socialism and labour unrest', in Brown (ed.), op. cit.

70 'Cultural decline of drapers', *Eastern Daily Press*, 10 January 1936.

71 'John Lewis and Company Limited', *The Economist*, 7 June 1930, pp. 1292–3.

72 '£10,000 gift for the hospital', *Bournemouth Daily Echo*, 24 October 1936.

73 A. Mond, *Industry and Politics*, London, 1927.

74 R. P. T. Davenport-Hines, 'Hirst, Hugo', in D. J. Jeremy and C. Shaw, *Dictionary of Business Biography*, London, 1985, quotation at p. 281.

75 A. Bullock, *The Life and Times of Ernest Bevin. Vol. I: Trade Union Leader 1881–1940*, London, 1960; Cantor, forthcoming, op. cit.

76 'Ideal employer robbed', *Westminster Record*, 10 June 1933, my emphasis.

77 'Mr. Selfridge's impressions', *Jersey Evening Post*, 22 June 1932.
78 Lord Nuffield, Sir Herbert Austin, Sir H. P. Croft, Col. J. Gretton, Sir Robert Horne: 'Joseph Chamberlain centenary', *The Times*, 16 June 1936.
79 Lord Croft, *My Life of Strife*, London, 1948.
80 Churchill College archives: Croft papers, CRFT 3/15, 3/16 and 3/17.
81 Sir Henry Page Croft, 'The British mandated territories', *Weekly Review*, 7 July 1938.
82 '£500,000 to combat rheumatic scourge', *Leader*, 26 June 1937; 'Empire war against rheumatism', *Overseas Daily Mail*, 7 November 1936; 'Empire-wide war on disease: call-to-arms in fight against rheumatism', *News of the World*, 26 December 1937.
83 'Two kinds of war: to destroy life and to destroy disease', *Manchester Guardian*, 27 January 1938; 'Two kinds of war', *Scotsman*, 27 January 1938.
84 'From warm beds to damp trenches', *Yorkshire Observer*, 20 December 1938.
85 'Britons free from nerves, says Duke of Gloucester', *Morning Advertiser*, 26 April 1939.
86 See for example the worries over the effect of commercial pressures on the spas, Cantor, 1990, op. cit.

INDEX